BIOLOGY AND ETHICS

(Proceedings of a Symposium held at the
Royal Geographical Society, London, on
26 and 27 September 1968)

Edited by

F. J. EBLING

Department of Zoology,
The University, Sheffield.
England

1969

Published for the
INSTITUTE OF BIOLOGY
by
ACADEMIC PRESS
LONDON and NEW YORK

ACADEMIC PRESS INC. (LONDON) LTD
Berkeley Square House
Berkeley Square
London, W1X 6BA

U.S. Edition published by
ACADEMIC PRESS INC.
111 Fifth Avenue
New York, New York 10003

Library of Congress Catalog Card Number: 77–92402
Standard Book Number: 12–229050–X

PRINTED IN GREAT BRITAIN BY
THE WHITEFRIARS PRESS LTD.
LONDON AND TONBRIDGE

Contributors

M. R. A. CHANCE, *Sub-department of Ethology, Uffculme Clinic, Birmingham, England*

C. A. CLARKE, *Nuffield Unit of Medical Genetics, University of Liverpool, Liverpool, England*

B. FOSS, *Department of Psychology, Bedford College, Regent's Park, London, England*

F. FRASER DARLING, *Conservation Foundation, Washington, D.C., U.S.A.*

J. E. HALL WILLIAMS, *London School of Economics, London, England*

J. H. HUMPHREY, *National Institute for Medical Research, Mill Hill, London, England*

R. P. MICHAEL, *Department of Psychiatry, Institute of Psychiatry, University of London, London, England*

B. MITCHELL, *Oriel College, Oxford, England*

A. S. PARKES, *Christ's College, Cambridge, England*

D. A. POND, *Department of Psychiatry, London Hospital Medical College, London, England*

M. POTTS, *Department of Anatomy, University of Cambridge, Cambridge, England*

A. RICHARDS, *University of Cambridge, Cambridge, England*

M. F. A. WOODRUFF, *Department of Surgical Science, University of Edinburgh, Edinburgh, Scotland*

Participants in the Discussion

H. J. BLACKHAM, *Twickenham, Middlesex, England*

W. B. BROUGHTON, *Sir John Cass College, London, England*

J. R. BUSVINE, *London School of Hygiene and Tropical Medicine, London, England*

A. V. S. de REUCK, *Centre for Analysis of Conflict, University College, London, England*

M. R. DOWDESWELL, *Melksham, Wiltshire, England*

C. B. GOODHART, *Department of Zoology, The University, Cambridge, England*

C. G. HEDÉN, *International Institute for Peace and Conflict Research, Stockholm, Sweden*

F. LE GROS CLARKE, *Cambridge, England*

E. MASON, *Edinburgh, Scotland*

N. W. MOORE, *Monk's Wood Experimental Station, Huntingdon, England*

P. N. O'DONOGHUE, *Royal Postgraduate Medical School, London, England*

T. B. POOLE, *Department of Zoology, University College, Aberystwyth, Wales*

J. W. S. PRINGLE, *Department of Zoology, The University, Oxford, England*

E. T. O. SLATER, *Psychiatric Genetics Research Unit, Maudsley Hospital, London, England*

B. TOWERS, *Jesus College, Cambridge, England*

H. V. WYATT, *Department of Biology, The University, Bradford, England*

Preface

I am grateful to the Institute of Biology for giving me the opportunity to convene the Symposium on "Biology and Ethics" and especially to its General Secretary, Mr. D. J. B. Copp, for his help in arranging the papers and compiling the discussion. I would like to thank the chairmen, contributors and participants on behalf of both the Institute of Biology and of myself, and also to express my gratitude to Academic Press.

The Introduction was not given at the Symposium but is an attempt to summarize and link some of the ideas of the contributors, as well as providing other relevant sources of information. I had intended to make an unbiased survey, but I found it impossible to write about the subject without expressing a personal attitude. I must, therefore, make it clear that my own views are in no sense to be attributed to the Institute of Biology.

JOHN EBLING

May, 1969
Symposium Convenor

Contents

Introduction

The concept of Natural Selection, by providing a feasible mechanism for evolution, irrevocably changed Man's beliefs about his own physical origin. The idea that he was but one product of a slow process of change over many millions of years, of the same stuff as apes and animalcules, and not a special creation in the image of God, at first seemed—in the Western world at least—to complete that demotion of man from the centre of his own universe which had been started by Galileo. Yet during the century following the publication of "The Origin of Species" evolution has widely replaced the various myths of creation.

In contrast, the impact of discoveries in comparative behaviour has yet to be felt. Philosophers may be less ready to make generalizations about human nature or to argue the semantics of value words than they were a few decades ago, but men in general continue to justify their institutions, beliefs, actions and motives by concepts of right and wrong that are as rigidly absolute as they are vaguely defined. Each, in the course of human events, accepts in varying degree duties and obligations; each assumes or demands rights. Each has an idea of Justice which is based on the firm principles of Equality before the law and Liberty of the subject, suitably tempered by considerations of Merit, especially when he himself is the beneficiary. Many are prepared, in theory at least, to apply such ideals to the whole of human society and, especially when their own interests are not obviously or immediately involved, even to urge others to do so in practice. Tolerance is recognised as a virtue, but disapproval by neighbours may still lead to ostracism; conscience may indeed be the final arbiter, but what the Church forbids remains heresy, and what is against the interest of the State may still be treason.

As men circle the moon in space capsules or transplant human hearts, many traditional values are, however, in decay or under attack. Democracy seems to be losing the confidence of the people, Communism is in schism, and the Pope's pronouncement is questioned by the faithful. Millions may starve among the emergent nations and even in the most prosperous societies the old appear neglected and the young are in revolt. Can biological science help in the understanding and perhaps in the solution of ethical problems?

The hypothesis of Natural Selection emphasized the constant competition for survival amongst individuals. Darwin (1872) stated this clearly, if not with undue succinctness, "A struggle for existence inevitably follows from the high rate at which all organic beings tend to increase. Every being, which during its natural lifetime produces several eggs or seeds, must suffer destruction during some period of its life, and during some season or occasional year, otherwise on the principle of geometrical increase, its numbers would quickly become so inordinately great that no country could support the product. Hence, as more individuals are produced than can possibly survive, there must in every case be a struggle for existence, either one individual with another of the same species, or with individuals of distinct species, or with the physical conditions of life. It is the doctrine of Malthus applied with manifold force to the whole animal and vegetable kingdoms; for in this case there can be no artificial increase of food, and no prudential restraint from marriage. Although some species may now be increasing, more or less rapidly, in numbers, all cannot do so, for the world would not hold them."

The major—and indeed magnificent—advances in biology since Darwin have been those which explain how variation, the substrate of natural selection, is produced at the levels of the chromosome and ultimately of the molecules of desoxyribose nucleic acid. It is clear, however, that over many areas of the animal kingdom the continuation of species depends more on the survival of social groups than of individuals. The group has two major selective advantages. It provides protection from enemies, for a predator can only concentrate on isolated prey and is confused by a mass such as a shoal of fish or a flock of birds, and it can be more efficient in the finding of food (Thorpe, 1965). It is thus at the group level that selection must operate and the way in which individuals interact in social groups becomes of paramount evolutionary importance. Moreover, since—as we shall see—the rapid and successful evolution of mammalian, and especially of human, societies depends upon the selection of behaviour patterns that are learned rather than inherited in the Mendelian sense, there is a whole field of biology of the greatest relevance to human affairs for which the reductionist approach is unprofitable if not irrelevant. It is surprising that post-Darwinian biology, while it has made such remarkable advances in elucidating the molecular basis for organic change, has been so slow in applying evolutionary ideas to the study of behaviour in highly organized animal societies, thus contributing to an understanding of the human estate. Some of the historical reasons for this are discussed by Michael Chance (p. 3, this book).

When in the course of evolution the survival of the group becomes more important to the species than the survival of the individual, it may be expected that two phenomena will make their appearance. On the one hand, organisms may co-operate rather than compete, as admirably discussed by Allee *et al.* (1950) and by Crook (1966); on the other, individuals may be sacrificed or sacrifice themselves for the sake of the group—the origin of altriusm. The necessity for such behavioural interactions has been argued *a priori*—though not without examples—by Wynne-Edwards (1962). If a species over exploits its environment so that no food resources remain available to it, the result must be disaster. Hence species must have homeostatic mechanisms to control their populations. For example, beavers fell trees in order to eat the tops. Since trees take many years to grow until they are cropable by beavers, it would clearly appear possible for any population of beavers to multiply to an extent which would destroy its own future resources. The optimum population which allows continued survival must be much below the possible maximum over a short term. Wynne-Edwards believes that territory, and the behavioural mechanisms which maintain it, play a major part in population homeostasis. One interesting example may be quoted, the prenuptial display or "lek" of game birds such as the black grouse. At the first light of dawn, in the spring or early summer, groups of five to twenty-five cock birds assemble on a customary ground and engage in ritualistic combat for the possession of territory. Only those males obtaining tenure of a display site subsequently mate. Similar behaviour is shown by an antelope known as the Uganda Kob (Ardrey, 1967). The predominance of territory has, however, been questioned. Critics have pointed out that the territorial thesis is based on selected examples and that many social groups either do not hold territories or, if they do, are flexible about its delineation and maintenance. Groups of chimpanzees, for example, wander over large home ranges and their behaviour is determined by competition for commodities rather than by territorial considerations.

Though the terms "co-operation" and "altruism" can be used to describe behavioural phenomena which contribute to the survival of the groups, how far are we justified in considering this the origin of ethical behaviour? To answer the question some attempt to define ethical behaviour must be made.

Human behaviour is said to be ethical or moral when it is "right" as opposed to "wrong", and a code of ethics is a system of what is considered "right" in any particular society. The nature of "rightness" and "wrongness" provides the material for the discipline of Ethics or Moral Philosophy. I have so far successfully—and deliberately—avoided any discussion of the meaning of such words and it is not necessary to the argument. By whatever philosophical contortions we attempt to derive or define our value judgements, the one important point is that ethical behaviour must involve a choice, as Basil Mitchell's admirable discussion (p. 37) makes clear. No moral approbation can be give to actions that are inevitable. In biological terms the nature of this choice appears to be clear; it arises from conflict between the mechanisms which promote survival of the organism and those which make for survival of the social group. One might expect these individual drives, such as hunger, sexual appetite and fear to have an instinctive component and their modification in the interests of society to involve learning. This division is not however very useful since all behaviour depends on both genetic and environmental factors, and moral choice may indeed arise from conflicts between acquired patterns of behaviour.

The drives to individual survival and reproduction may be equated with the "id" of Freud, the great subconscious appetite—with the sexual urge paramount—striving for satisfaction. The "ego" and the "super-ego"—more or less equivalent to conscience—which Freud differentiates from it represent the mechanisms which modify and control the instincts to accommodate the demands of the external world. The ego and super-ego are not to be thought of as conscious mediators applying ethical codes; only a part of our ethical behaviour passes through the channels of consciousness.

How and when can ethical behaviour be considered to have arisen in evolution? Though in bird behaviour we may find models which demonstrate the selective advantage of "altruism", we must be careful about regarding this as an ethical phenomenon. It is true that birds do learn; song is handed down from generation to generation by imitation and local dialects can develop, and the geographical spread by learning of other behavioural traits has been recorded (see Thorpe, 1965). But bird behaviour is largely genetically programmed. Similarly, we must agree with Mitchell (p. 37) that the "bravery" of soldier ants is not an action calling for moral assessment of any kind.

For the origin of behaviour that is "ethical" in the sense of involving "choice" or conflict we may look amongst the mammals and especially amongst those socially organized sub-human primates, as described by Chance (p. 3). Examples of co-operation in such societies have been considered (see Crook, 1966), but it is doubtful how many of them can be cited as examples of altruism; some appear more like exploitation. Chimpanzees can learn to co-operate in solving problems and will share food, though dominant animals always profit the most by these operations. However, that animals can learn to subjugate individual appetites has been nicely demonstrated (Solomon *et al.*, 1968, referred to by Foss p. 33). Solomon was able to train puppies not to eat certain foods by cuffing them with a folded newspaper either as they approached the food or after they had eaten some. After the first procedure, puppies refrained from taking the food even in the absence of surveillance or immediate threat, as if they had developed "consciences". That a cultural habit can become initiated and spread has been experimentally shown in macaque colonies (Myiadi, 1959). Monkeys were offered paper wrapped caramels, and at first these were refused. Gradually they were accepted and unwrapped by young monkeys, but only when they were not watched or corrected by adults. However, the habit slowly spread, even to the mothers and finally to the males.

Man occupies a unique position because in the course of his evolution his ethical behaviour becomes conceptualized and codified. Of specu- lation about the possible origin of primitive ethical concepts, Thorpe (1965) has written, "This is a path along which pitfalls of every kind abound; as is I think shown only too clearly by many previous specu- lations on the subject, even those emanating from the most learned. It seems safe to say that we shall never know more than a tiny fraction of the facts which would be necessary to arrive at anything like a coherent and convincing account".

It is difficult not to share Thorpe's caution. The problem is bound up with the evolution of, on the one hand language and the ability to conceive of and communicate abstractions, and on the other religion— the awareness of and ritualized communication with the organic and cosmic universe. If, however, we accept that ethical behaviour precedes, rather than proceeds from, the emergence of ethical concepts, con- ceptualization falls into perspective as only one—albeit important— development in an evolutionary sequence that as a whole can properly be studied by comparative methods.

Primitive human communities share with animal societies the acceptance of hierarchies which involve privileges over food and rights over territory. But status obligations are generally handed on and not continually established anew by contest. Indeed, behaviour as a whole —as Audrey Richards makes clear (p. 23)—is based on a transmitted memory of the past—a culture handed from generation to generation. The ethical systems of closed societies differ so widely that one cannot dispute the view of Leach (1967) that there are no universal rules of morality except, perhaps, those forbidding mother-son incest. How- ever, Richards points out that the areas of behaviour governed by such rules hardly vary at all from culture to culture. In particular, primitive peoples have elaborate rules of mating and kinship which are designed to enlarge and stabilize the community. The mating rules serve not to prevent inbreeding but to promote alliances, the orderly passage of property and the control of children, and to reduce the risk of conflicts.

The primitive community is concerned solely with behaviour within its own confines. The next stage in the development of human culture is the conceptualization of principles for more general application—the transition from the "closed" society to the "open" one. This, according to Mitchell (p. 37), required the rise of critical and creative judgement on the part of the individual. The spread of the great religions, of which Christianity is discussed because it is an essential part of our own history, can be viewed as part of this process. "Socrates and Jesus do not simply internalize the codes of their own society; they criticize them in the name of an ideal society", writes Mitchell. From the evolutionary viewpoint the transition from closed to open societies is important. In the closed society, selective forces operate alike on moral code and social community. The code is not for export; society and code flourish—or perish—together. The "open" morality, on the other hand, transcends any particular society; it aims to create a universal ideal society. For Mitchell this jump is too big to explain in evolutionary language. "Even if the concept of natural selection can be stretched far enough to account for the moral codes of closed societies, it cannot be made to cover 'open morality'." Mitchell argues that whether or not natural selection can produce a being capable of moral reflection, the values which that being recognizes are not themselves a product of natural selection, but of conscious thought. Mitchell's difficulties recall some earlier ones of Thorpe (1965). On Pantin's idea that the success of natural selection depended on the fact that "the Universe is such that the right materials are available and appropriate engineering solutions are possible", Thorpe commented "But this fitness of the conditions of existence would have to account for such remarkable features as the emergence of individual consciousness, features which seem to elude explanation on this basis alone—even granting that the unique properties of carbon, hydrogen and oxygen are fully accounted for in physical terms".

Is it, however, necessary to propose that moral values themselves are a product of natural selection, any more than the Mona Lisa, Hamlet, or Beethoven's Ninth Symphony? Could it be that, once the ability to create and manipulate abstractions has been evolved and applied to the analysis of behaviour, moral precepts become the substrate of 'selection' rather than its result—the creative mutations of cultural evolution? In the change from the closed to open ethical system, 'selection' no longer operates on the group, but on the system itself. Thus the growth—or decay—of religious or political systems, Christianity, Islam—or Communism—might be seen neither as a result of historical accident or divine intervention, nor of the zeal of missionaries or the force of arms, but of the social advantages, in the widest sense, conferred by them.

Human beings seem to have a remarkable aptitude for acquiring moral attitudes, which sometimes seems to exceed their capacity for intelligent behaviour. Stated attitudes are not, of course, necessarily correlated with behaviour; in Foss's words (p. 15), "The relation between saying and doing is not high". How do ethical feelings arise in the development of the individual?

Foss suggests that three main mechanisms may be involved in learning to conform and maintaining conformity. Firstly, people seek tangible rewards, social approbation, or the more subtle pleasures of belonging to groups which share common tastes, habits, jargon, or even a common object of admiration or dislike. Secondly, they desire to avoid punishment, of which social isolation—loneliness—is one of the most potent and which may include less obvious forms such as ridicule. Thirdly, they may imitate. A child may come to conform by modelling himself on others, at first on someone close to and loved by him and later on members of social groups which he joins.

Social approval and disapproval continue to influence people throughout their lives, but the avoidance of non-moral behaviour depends also on an internal control—or conscience—which operates independently of external comment. Experimental evidence from puppies and studies of human delinquency both seem to confirm a commonly held, indeed traditional, view that conscience develops early in childhood and is best fostered by a combination of affection and discipline; psychological deterrence—the threatened withdrawal of affection—is more effective than aggressive verbal and physical punishments.

Before the age of eight a child can understand and accept the idea of strict liability for damage caused by his actions. Rules are strict and almost mythically god-given—to quote Foss—and the breaking of them requires punishment. Not until about the age of ten does the child appreciate that wrong doing must imply intent, or that rules are intended to be socially beneficial and can be changed by mutual consent.

Conscience provides an internal mechanism which suppresses desires to break the ethical code, even when this can be done without detection or external disapproval. The breaking of the code, or urges to break it, result in conflict which manifests itself as feelings of guilt. However, as Desmond Pond (p. 55) shows, the emotional state of guilt can dominate people who lead blameless lives, and yet in others it may be lacking even before, during or after the commission of serious crimes. The development of a sense of guilt is clearly associated with, and may give some insight into, the origin of conscience. There is little doubt that it starts in the early months of life; a "paralysing and irrational" sense of guilt can be found early on in children. Indeed it is important to ensure that guilty feelings do not become disastrously attached to ethically neutral behavioural traits, such as masturbation. For an entertaining account of such superfluous guilts—the overspill of the conscience mechanism—the reader is referred to Alex Comfort's book "The Anxiety Makers" (1967).

In the legal sense, guilt at first sight appears to be an objective state. A person is guilty—whether or not they feel any sense of guilt—if they are proved to have committed an offence against the law. With some exceptions, however, guilt under British law requires not only the commission of an illegal act but that the person committing it shall fulfil a number of criteria of responsibility which, as Hall Williams (p. 45) points out, are mainly psychological in character. In legal language guilt requires not only *actus reas*—the criminal act, but *mens rea*—the guilty mind. Thus in common law, insanity of such a degree that the defendant did not know his action was wrong, infancy, i.e. being under the age of ten, and coercion are among several possible legitimate defences. In short, the attitude of common law is much the same as that of the moral philosopher; it is not the social consequence of the act but the criminal intent which is paramount; wrong doing can only arise as a deliberate act after a free choice.

Accepting these criteria, punishment logically would appear to be a retribution for breaking the ethical code. The judicial homily expresses the abhorrence not only of current society but of tradition, and the judge's stricture is an expression of his own feelings of guilt as he identifies himself with the defendant—a theme brilliantly exploited in a play by the lawyer and playwright, John Mortimer (1967). For the prisoner, punishment supposedly provides expiation; while it is doubtful how many old prison hands would accept this thesis, the idea seems to be nicely expressed in the phrase used by a guilty defendant when he "asks for (so many) other offences to be taken into consideration", thus insuring himself against further convictions and penalties.

The common law approach to criminal responsibility clearly represents a valuable bed rock of justice. In a number of ways, however, the law is too conservative to meet either the requirements of our complex society or the aspirations of liberal penologists, and traditional concepts have been or are being modified. These questions are admirably discussed by Hall Williams (p. 45), but I draw attention to some of the difficulties here because they throw light as a whole on the function of ethics in society.

On the one hand, some legislation appears more to reflect archaic feelings of guilt than serve any useful purpose. This is particularly so in relation to sexual offences, such as homosexual behaviour, discussed by Richard Michael (p. 67), and prostitution, of which Wayland Young (1965) has written "In our society now, prostitution is specialized, mercenary, and reprobated. We confine the function to individual women who become a class apart. . . . . . We pay them for exercising their function. We also despise and penalize them. . . . We project on the prostitute our own guilty desires, because our accepted values declare us low and beastly when we go to her, we feel that she is herself low and beastly".

On the other hand, during the last hundred years or so, a series of offences have been created by statute, in order to serve particular social or economic policies, which do not require guilty intent; the defendant is "strictly liable". Such legislation is often criticized, particularly when a conviction appears to transgress against a traditional idea of justice. Strict liability seems to have prevailed in early societies, and ontogenetically it can be appreciated by the child before the idea of intent; both these facts appear to support the view of Hall Williams that legislation of this type represents a severe setback for civilized legal ideals. At the same time, in some activities the border lines between recklessness, negligence and pure accident are not always easy to determine and there are pressures to increase the areas of strict liability. It is, for example, often claimed that strict liability for damage caused by motor cars would reduce the number of accidents.

Two further problems, namely the limits of responsibility and the aim of punishment, are related to each other. No one denies that an imbecile or a young child is not responsible for his actions. It is, nevertheless, necessary for society to protect itself from or desirable to provide for the care of an offender; the law functions not solely to bring retribution to wrongdoers but to protect society and reform the offender. The solutions to the legal dilemma seem, in the light of the doctrine of *mens rea*, to be both illogical and sensible. The illogicality is nicely seen in the verdict "Guilty, but insane", when obviously an insane person cannot have guilty intent and cannot, therefore, be deserving of punishment. Society is protected and—we hope—the prisoner is treated by detaining him during Her Majesty's pleasure at a mental hospital. Similarly, a plea of diminished responsibility, applicable only to murder, is not a defence against conviction, but can only mitigate the penalty. Further inroads into the idea of responsibility, which are likely to follow from an increased understanding of the psychology and physiology of personality disorders, may well be accommodated in a similar way.

The law is thus a compromise between the dictates of tradition, the current demands of society embodied in statute, and the aspirations of reformers. The aim of punishment, stated by Hall Williams, is an amalgam of retribution, deterrence and reform; the protection of society may be added.

The idea of an evolutionary approach to ethics is, of course, by no means new. Traditional theological or metaphysical theories have generally held that moral truths are universal, revealed by intuition, and in accord with the absolute will of God, the perfect function of some essential nature of man or, as implied in the idea of Natural Law due to Thomas Aquinas, with both in harmony together. In contrast, naturalistic philosophers have sought, not always without difficulty, to define ethical values using the same kinds of criteria as are used for scientific concepts.

How can a virtuous act be described in these terms? The early naturalistic philosophers, such as Epicurus in about 300 B.C., saw the pursuit of happiness as the moral aim of life; each person *ought* to act to further his own pleasures. In the nineteenth century, the English philosophers, Jeremy Bentham (1748-1832) and John Stuart Mill (1806-1873) developed the more universally acceptable proposition that rightness is a quality characteristic of acts which produce the greatest happiness for the greatest number, an ethical system usually known as "utilitarianism". The more recent philosophy of "pragmatism" which defines the good as that which promotes social advance by resolving conflicts which impede it, is clearly in the mainstream of naturalistic ethics.

The view that ethical behaviour and ethical ideas have evolved was a natural development of the utilitarian philosophy as well as of Darwin's theory of Natural Selection. Herbert Spencer first put forward such an evolutionary idea (later developed into "The Data of Ethics", 1879), maintaining that 'we must interpret the more developed by the less developed', even before publication of "The Origin of Species". Darwin (1871) himself experienced some difficulty in seeing why natural selection should lead to higher moral standards: "It is extremely doubtful whether the offspring of the more sympathetic and benevolent parents, or of those who were the most faithful to their comrades, would be reared in greater numbers than the children of selfish and treacherous parents belonging to the same tribe". Thomas Henry Huxley was clearly opposed to intuitional theories of ethics and believed moral sentiments to have originated "in the same way as other natural phenomena by a process of evolution". But, as Julian Huxley (1947) has pointed out, T. H. Huxley seems nevertheless to have accepted the ethical values of his time as self-evident, so that he uses terms like *good* and *evil* without any attempt at definition, and (see Waddington, 1942), far from accepting that social change must be good, he was morally outraged by what he believed to be the character of the cosmic process—the "gladiatorial theory of existence". "Let us understand once and for all", wrote Huxley, "that the ethical progress of society depends, not on imitating the cosmic process, still less in running away from it, but in combating it". The rise of evolutionary ethics and the contributions of Herbert Spencer, Charles Darwin, T. H. Huxley and others has been splendidly discussed elsewhere by Julian Huxley (1947).

More recently, Waddington (1942) and Julian Huxley (1947) have put forward versions of the evolutionary argument. For Waddington, the question at issue is "whether the ethical beliefs which form part of the super-ego are injected into the individual apart from and independently of his experience of the material world, or whether they are formed by the interaction of the personality and the world; there cannot be any question of the super-ego being impressed by external circumstances on to a merely receptive and featureless individual". Waddington continues, "The answer which I am urging is that the situation is actually parallel to that with which we are familar in genetics; all characters are, as Goodrich put it, both inherited and acquired; they are products of the interaction between the genes, which we usually consider internal, and the equally necessary factors, such as oxygen, nourishment, etc. which we usually consider external. Strictly speaking, one cannot say that the propositions of ethics arise from the experience of external, as opposed to internal, connexions; their origin is that the observation the world is such, and the personality is such, that the individual must follow certain rules". Waddington concludes, "It is, then, finally clear that science is in a position to make a contribution to ethics, since ethics is based on facts of the kind with which science deals. And the nature of science's contribution is also clear; it is the revelation of the nature, the character and direction of the evolutionary process in the world as a whole, and the elucidation of the consequences, in relation to that direction, of the various courses of human action".

With equal clarity, Julian Huxley (1947) has stated that all purely intuitive theories of ethics can be ruled out because of advances in psychology which show how the precursor of conscience develops. He has christened this precursor the "proto-ethical" mechanism. "All that the child inherits is a capacity for building up what we have called the proto-ethical mechanism, and even that will not take place in all circumstances. Its "intuitions" as to what constitutes right or wrong are derived from its environment, largely mediated through its mother". The proto-ethical mechanism can, indeed, go severely wrong. Huxley recognises that unjust or stupid treatment of the child can superimpose an excessive load of guilt which may lead to an irrational sense of unworthiness or even of self-hatred. The conscience can set up no claim to absolute authority; such claims are dangerous since those who make them are likely to be victims of a distorted and hyperactive conscience. But Huxley does not deny the importance of conscience: "In so far as the proto-ethical mechanism is itself undistorted and its feeling of rightness reflects, albeit in embryonic form, a morality that is objectively right, it can then be developed by reason and aspiration into a conscience which will be an indispensable moral guide".

Lack (1957) is among biologists who have expressed disagreement with Waddington and Huxley. He believes that it is impossible to justify high moral standards or abstract truths from the evolutionary process. He states that the claim of Darwinism that man has evolved wholly by natural means is philosophical, not scientific, and has thus acquired a spurious authority. He proceeds to argue that "if an essential part of human nature lies outside the terms of reference of science, then since all natural phenomena can be studied scientifically, it would appear to follow that man has not evolved wholly by natural means. If, on the other hand, man evolved wholly by natural means, then all human nature should be interpretable in scientific terms, which would seem to make individual responsibility an illusion, high moral standards a mistake, and intellectual conclusions untrustworthy". Lack's argument seems to be related to the contention of G. E. Moore (1903), in his 'Principia Ethica', that it is a naturalistic fallacy to attempt to identify moral notions, such as 'good', which are unique and non-natural, with non-moral notions, and his conclusion that ethics cannot therefore be reduced to or derived from natural science.

Thorpe (1965), has similarly expressed strong disagreement with the "assumption implicit in much of Waddington's argument that because man evolved as a physical being he cannot then know any other realms of existence. The animal mind is undoubtedly an efficient instrument for carrying out the essential biological activities; and in so

far as man's mind is of the same class of organization, the same thing
can be said of the human mind. But I for one should react strongly
against any suggestion that we are, let alone must ever remain, in our
mental qualities, animals and nothing more". This again is a statement
of conviction rather than an argued refutation. Yet Thorpe is by no
means hostile to the evolutionary idea, and he seems prepared even to
apply it to religion; but his views reveal a constant search for design in
the initiation and course of evolution. He is particularly concerned
with the origin of what he calls 'spirituality'—the quality that manifests
itself in religious awareness and ritual—and its relation to the origin of
ethical beliefs. One other idea of Thorpe's is of particular interest,
namely that "progress in human society involves increasing versatility
of individuals and increasing diversity of individuals so long as they
are harmoniously adapted to one another", a paraphase of Thoday's
(1958) remark that "biological progress not only involves increasing
versatility of individual species but also increasing diversity of species
harmoniously adapted to one another". Thorpe argues from this that
the development of tolerance of versatility and diversity is perhaps the
most important single factor permitting and encouraging social
progress.

The argument that evolutionary theories must be fallacious because
value judgements are unique in that they cannot be established by
inference can be profitably examined further by a study of Bertrand
Russell (1947). Russell, who admits to having been more influenced by
Moore than by any other single philosopher, appears to accept his
theory of value. "Ethics differs from science in the fact that its fundamental data are feelings and emotions, not precepts" he writes, and he
points out that ethical judgements should be enunciated in the imperative mood; the injunction "thou shalt love thy neighbour as thyself"
is a pure ethical sentence which "clearly cannot be proved or disproved
merely by amassing facts". But Russell then proceeds to "attempt to
set forth an undogmatic ethic and apply it to political problems" by
arguments which are very similar to those of Huxley, although they
are cloaked in somewhat different language. "Man, like other animals,"
according to Russell, "is filled with impulses and passions which, on the
whole, ministered to survival while man was emerging. But his intelligence has shown him that his passions are often self-defeating. . . Ethics
and moral codes are necessary to man because of the conflict between
intelligence and impulse. Given intelligence only, or impulse only,
there would be no place for ethics."

Russell is clear that the main purpose of morals is to promote
behaviour serving the interests of the group and not merely of the

individual. "I think that the 'objectively right' act is that which best serves the interest of the group that is regarded as ethically dominant". But what is an "ethically dominant group"? "The difficulty" says Russell, "is that this group will be differently defined by different people and in different circumstances". He goes on to admit that there is no theoretical ground for preferring one group to another. The admission is, however, not a confession of failure but the starting point from which he argues that a stable world society can be constructed on scientific principles, given certain conditions.

The arguments in support of a purely naturalistic theory of ethics, and the objections to it, may now be summarized. There is a measure of agreement amongst contributors to the symposium, and support from other biological authors, that behaviour which serves the interests of the group and may thus conflict with the desires of the individual, is the result of and subject to an evolutionary process. Such behaviour is "inherited" and becomes to some extent built into each individual through the "conscience" mechanism and it is reinforced and maintained in society by a range of devices from informal sanctions to the formal threat of the law.

The objections to the evolutionary view seem to centre around the "naturalistic fallacy", the idea that value judgements cannot be identified with or derived from non-moral notions which describe phenomena, and thus moral notions cannot be evolved. Surely, however, it is an "intuitive fallacy" to suppose that, because it is possible to create such moral abstractions and utilize them as instructions for social behaviour, the system becomes exempted from scientific examination? Because ethical instructions can be conceptualized and form part of language does not give such abstractions an existence which is independent of the situations to which they are directed or of the experience on which they are based.

The proposed model is, nevertheless, much too simple. Modern society is not monolithic but plural; within any society are many smaller groups such as religious organizations, political parties or even professional organizations, which have their own codes, virtues, loyalties and injunctions to behaviour. Though there is common agreement about major ethical issues throughout large areas of the world, every group, from church to children's 'gang' exhibits its own variations. Conflicting systems may co-exist or be partially reconciled and a single individual may adhere to more than one system and may be guided by different codes according to circumstance. A gentleman's word is his bond and he always tells the truth unless it be in defence of a lady's honour; yet a minister of the crown may be required not to tell the whole truth if national security demands, but be forced to resign if he lies about his sexual relationships.

Ethical notions are not only injunctions from society to its members, they are also instructions from individuals to society. Each individual, each component group, endeavours to influence the mores of the larger open society, national and international, of which it forms a part. It is thus impossible to dissociate ethics from politics. The political machinery provides the formal mediation between the individual and society. On the one hand, individuals elect and try to influence their leaders; on the other, the state requires conformity by the electors; thus a political election is as much a ritualistic exercise for the integration of society as a procedure for deciding who shall govern. But the democratic process is only part of the interaction, which takes place at many levels and through every available medium of communication. Social groups are integrated by mechanisms as widely different as religious worship, football matches and public demonstrations, and both state and individual are subject to a barrage of persuasion from pressure groups—pope and priest, press barons and advertising agents.

This field is far too wide to be covered in our symposium and we have no sociological or political contributors. But the link between biology and sociology is investigated by Michael Chance, who is particularly concerned with the way leaders are chosen. Can the study of animal behaviour replace mythical and traditional ways of thinking about human affairs as Chance suggests? He points out that many sub-human primate societies, for example, gorillas, chimpanzees and baboons, as well as simple human ones, are centripetally organized around dominant males who achieve their position by display potential. When danger threatens, individuals run to their overlords for protection. The rise of demagogues or dictators in times of social unrest offers a striking human parallel. The problem is to utilize intelligent judgement to establish and brief competent authority.

If ethical behaviour is evolved and if the creative moral injunctions that relate to it persist when they promote the biological survival of society, can ethical directives have any goal? In the absence of any reference to absolute authority, what guarantee is there that such directives will be efficacious? The answer must be that there is no such guarantee. But this is far from saying that there can be no criteria for the formulation of moral injunctions. The whole of human history and experience is available as a basis for them. The essence of evolutionary processes is that change occurs because a changing environment favours the survival of variations within an already evolved pattern. Thus creative ethical injunctions must neither remain hidebound to superstition or to beliefs which have served a totally different society, nor are they likely to endure if they completely reject tradition. Can one deny that ethical innovators will benefit from the understanding which comes from increased knowledge of human behaviour and human ecology? Or, knowing that time may prove them wrong, that they will approach the problem with any less humility than purely intuitive philosophers?

In this light contributors to the symposium proceed to discuss some of the main ethical problems of our time. Should man take for granted a 'right' to unlimited reproduction and unlimited exploitation of the natural world, regardless either of other species or of the needs of human posterity? In primitive cultures there is a rudimentary sense of reciprocation to the environment, as when an Athabascan Indian asks forgiveness of the bear he is about to hunt and kill and is thus philosophically conscious of his own ecological situation. Agricultural and industrial societies have become vastly more ruthless with disastrous results too well known to need cataloguing. The idea of conservation, regarded by some as no more than sentimental, and of population control (p. 109), regarded by others as an interference with natural law, are rational attempts to put the development of man back into a biological context and are proper matters of ethical concern.

Modern scientific discoveries present even more difficult problems for which there are no clear ethical precedents in traditional attitudes. To what extent should life be prolonged by artificial machinery, when no hope of conscious recovery remains? What degree of suffering should a doctor be prepared to inflict on patients in the hope of prolonging life? Should the conception or gestation of children who will have no chance of normal life or who carry a high genetic risk of painful and early death be permitted? Whatever we believe about the source and inspiration of ethical injunctions it is not possible to baulk these issues. Such problems of a medical nature have been debated elsewhere (Royal Society of Medicine, 1967; Wolstenholme and O'Connor, 1966) and form only a small though important part of our symposium. But pure scientists also face moral issues for which the responsibility cannot be passed to society at large and towards which traditional injunctions are equivocal. Have scientists, for example, a duty to place every means of military destruction at the disposal of their governments—or have they a clear responsibility to refuse to develop methods of genocide? If our symposium can reach decision over little and must omit much, we cannot escape from the problems it presents.

MAY 1969   JOHN EBLING

REFERENCES

Allee, W. C., Emerson, A. E., Park, O., Park, T. and Schmidt, K. P. (1950). "Principles of Animal Ecology". W. B. Saunders, Philadelphia and London.

Ardrey, R. (1967). "The Territorial Imperative". Collins, London.

Comfort, A. (1967). "The Anxiety Makers". Thomas Nelson and Sons, London.

Crook, J. H. (1966). Co-operation in Primates. *Eugenics Rev.* **58,** 63-70.

Darwin, C. (1871). "The Descent of Man". London.

Darwin, C. (1872). "On The Origin of Species". Sixth edition. London.

Huxley, T. H. and Huxley, J. (1947). "Evolution and Ethics 1893-1943". Pilot Press, London.

Lack, D. (1957). "Evolutionary Theory and Christian Belief". Methuen, London.

Leach, E. (1967). "A Runaway World". B.B.C. Reith Lectures, London.

Moore, G. E. (1903). "Principia Ethica". University Press, Cambridge.

Mortimer, J. (1967). "The Judge". Methuen, London.

Myiadi, D. (1959). "On some new habits and their propagation in Japanese monkey groups". Proc. 15th Int. Congr. Zool. London, 875.

Royal Society of Medicine (1967). The Cost of Life. *Proc. R. Soc. Med.* **60,** 1195-1246.

Russell, B. (1954). "Human Society in Ethics and Politics". George Allen and Unwin, London.

Solomon, R. L., Turner, L. H. and Lessac, M. S. (1968). Some effects of the delay of punishment on resistance to temptation in dogs. *J. Personality Soc. Psychol.*, **8,** 233-238.

Spencer, H. (1879). "The Data of Ethics". London.

Thoday, J. M. (1958). Natural Selection and Biological Progress. *In* "A Century of Darwin" (ed. Barnett, S. A.), 313-333. Heinemann, London.

Thorpe, W. H. (1965). "Science, Man and Morals". Methuen, London.

Waddington, C. H. (1942). "Science and Ethics". George Allen and Unwin, London.

Wolstenholme, G. E. W. and O'Connor, M. (1966). Eds. "Ethics in Medical Progress: with special reference to Transplantation." J. and A. Churchill, London.

Wynne-Edwards, V. C. (1926). "Animal Dispersion in relation to Social Behaviour". Oliver and Boyd, Edinburgh and London.

Young, W. (1965). "Eros Denied". Weidenfeld and Nicolson, London.

Chairmen of the Sessions

Dr. C. E. Ford

Professor J. W. S. Pringle

N. W. Pirie

Dr. E. T. O. Slater

Towards the Biological Definition of Ethics

M. R. A. CHANCE

Sub-department of Ethology, Uffculme Clinic,
Birmingham, England

It is the purpose of this article to construct a behavioural model for ethics. Ethics are injunctions to action, and social action in particular, given by a group or society to its members, by one individual to another, and from one individual to himself (his conscience), and it will be argued, from an individual to society.

It will be argued that injunctions accepted by the individual from the group or from another individual in our present society do not involve the same types of social activity as when the individual attempts to bring about changes in society. The forms which individual initiative in changing society must take, if democracy is to advance, need more understanding. The mores of a society define types of behaviour appropriate to specific occasions, and in simple societies obedience to authority is synonymous with conformity with these mores, but in a democracy (being the articulate form of a pluralistic society), the individuals are providing injunctions for social action through a number of different sub-groups, some of which influence government, or are intended to set the limits or influence the direction of government action. Therefore, living in a democracy, we need to know how far individuals are capable of changing the direction of human affairs. Democrats also believe that, in general, intelligent solutions of problems are preferable to what are usually described as "emotional" solutions; therefore we need to know what behavioural features promote intelligent suggestions for action to arise from the society and how they can influence the selection of leaders. The role of biology, and ethology in particular, in this process will have to be discussed.

It is clear from the recent history of Europe that individuals who are far from being directed by intelligence in their behaviour can rise to the top of society and practically destroy it. This was evident in the case of Hitler, but few people are aware that the same processes lead to a large number of individuals rising to the top of society who possess many of the characteristics that were possessed by Hitler. In his book, "A Pattern of Rulers", Francis Williams has argued cogently that we

are not in control of the process which leads to the emergence of leaders
in a democracy, as, on his evidence, many of the leaders of the democratic society of the 1930's showed psychotic or neurotic characteristics
which amounted to incompetence in their profession, and they were as
much responsible for the rise of Hitler as were the incompetent
democrats of the Weimar republic. In the circumstances, I think it is
true to say that a present mood of disillusionment with democratic
procedures is not unfounded, since although much has been learned
since the 1930's, science has had little impact on the structure of
democracy or the way to promote the election of competent leaders.
In the meanwhile, what has biology been up to?—certainly not much
that can help, and a great deal that makes man's problems even
greater. As Abraham Maslow has said: "A biologist will soon have the
power to control and manipulate our genes, our own nervous system,
the hormones, the general chemistry of the body and evolution itself.
This raises even more urgently the question of what is desirable and
what is undesirable in the human being"—even as is being discussed
in this book—"the question of which persons shall live, reproduce and
which shall not. How will the biologist judge—how will they select
—on what criteria? Have they even considered the problem? If not
biologists, who else?", and he continues, *We have not yet fully defined
the nature of the human species.*" This is about the best statement yet
about the contribution that biologists should make to the solution of
these human problems (not forgetting that political control is a deciding
factor in the consideration of these problems), but they are under a
misapprehension if they think they can do this without knowing first of
all what is the structure of behaviour. As I look down the list of
contributors, I note that the Institute of Biology is not in a position to
draw on many biologists for assistance on the subject of the book
because biologists have made singularly little attempt to contribute
to these fields of investigation, and psychology and anthropology are
not, as yet, biologically based disciplines. Biologists, however, still
rely on traditional methods of thinking about ethics, and naturally
enough, therefore, find themselves at loggerheads with each other on
specific issues, because as well as being biologists they are members of
different sub-groups of our pluralistic society. Biologists will therefore
not be able to make a uniquely biological contribution to the solution
of ethical problems until they are able to think about the direction of
man's evolution, and this means bringing the study of every aspect of
modern man within the compass of biological studies.

This has not yet been done because, historically, the position in
which we are now represents the last stage in a process in which man

attempted to bring intellectual order into the universe around him and to shape his ideas on an appreciation of reality. Remarkably enough, he started with the furthest objects of his vision, the stars in the sky, and, having discovered for himself the order of their motions 3,000 years ago in ancient Sumeria, proceeded to bring his understanding down to earth in Greek science. The nearest thing to himself and the last to be scientifically investigated is his own nature.

Out of this process also came the early development of astronomy, physics and chemistry as sciences with well-established disciplines and theoretical foundations. The early growth of these sciences has subsequently influenced our approach to our own nature more than we are aware of. This has led to the present position, in which biology is infiltrated and almost dominated by the philosophy of reductionism, namely the belief that biological investigation leads to an explanation of biological phenomena only if sought in terms of physics, chemistry and mathematics. This means that when biologists want to investigate the nature of human behaviour it is done by utilizing neuro-physiological and biochemical concepts in an attempt to explain the phenomenon of behaviour without previously having described the phenomenon itself, or knowing anything about the forms of the behaviour as revealed by social anthropologists and ethologists. As a biologist surveying the scene at the present time, I am surprised to discover how much this process has been influencing my own thought, so that only at the age of fifty have I been able to recognize the logical thing for biologists to have done following the publication of "The Origin of Species" would have been to investigate the link between the organism and its environment; this would have been to describe and investigate animal and human behaviour. Behaviour is the link between the organism and its environment and can ultimately give us greater insight into the process that Darwin outlined, yet this has not been done until ethology, the latest development of the behavioural sciences, came on to the scene.

There are two ways in which earlier discussions of biology and ethics seem to me to have gone into a *cul-de-sac*. The first is adequately discussed and largely disposed of by Waddington in Chapter 8 of his "Ethical Animal", published in 1960, when he points out that if one opens any book of the present day "dealing with epistomology or the general problems of philosophy, you will find a discussion of the theory of relativity, the quantum theory, the indeterminacy principle and so on", and he comments that these, "though exceedingly important matters, are, one would have thought, somewhat remote from the general activities of human beings except in the very special field of quantitative analysis of behaviour of material bodies". Man is, as he says, a biological entity. It is only in his most generalized characteristics which he shares with sticks and stones that he is part of the subject matter of physics and chemistry. If we grant the substance of his argument and admit at once that biochemists have something to say on these matters in biology one can see now that the concern with whether or not these were suitable analogues upon which to explain human behaviour arose out of the predominantly reductionist philosophy that dominates biology. The second way is that which affirms that because evolution has taken place, we too are evolving, and so there must be an evolutionary direction in which we are proceeding, and this argument has been stated very profusely by Julian Huxley and again by Waddington. I sympathize with the sentiments that are expressed, but I find it extremely difficult to sympathize with the arguments, since most of these are confused by what are largely traditional ways of thinking.

Man is, as we know, largely dominated by the traditions of thought which he inherits from previous generations, and while this has undoubtedly served him immensely well in the immediate past, and has indeed been related to the differentiation of different languages and cultures, it largely reflects the situation today in which there are a number of national sub-groups of humanity competing with each other for survival, and capable, if the process gets out of hand, of destroying the species. I am not, therefore, so enamoured of the current view that man's outstanding quality is his creation of different traditions. Much more important would seem to be how to get away from the concepts that have, in fact, been derived from the use of traditional methods of thought and to try to define, from the study of the relevant biological material, what are the likely possible functions of ethical principles.

What we are attempting to do in the science of ethology is to replace mythical and traditional ways of thinking about behaviour with ways better modelled on reality, by first of all describing behaviour and the structure that can only then be properly investigated. Since we have not yet done this, this is the reason why we are in no position as biologists to contribute essentially to the problems discussed at this symposium. One of the major injunctions from this analysis is that it is incumbent on biologists to put their house in order by immediately reallocating resources within biology to redress the imbalance of information which is influencing man's awareness of himself from biology. At least one per cent of all biological researches should be switched to ethology immediately—this is an injunction if ever there was one. Clearly it needs justifying and I intend to communicate, from the inadequate ethological evidence already available, one probable biological dimension in which ethological principles will be needed to change human behaviour in a way appropriate to our present state of evolution towards an emergent world society.

This, as I have pointed out, can only be done with the relevant knowledge which is obtained from ethology, for ethological studies are, first of all, derived from the description of behaviour, which gives us an opportunity of discovering the properties and structure of behaviour. This concept, that behaviour has a structure, is however so new that few ethologists themselves are fully aware that it is a statement of fact about their work.

An ethic is simply a statement in language of the way in which it would be desirable to change behaviour in a given direction. The question therefore arises in what direction is behaviour changeable? This divides itself into two categories; what changes are possible in the adult human being and what in ontogeny? Space does not permit me to do more than state categorically certain important ethological discoveries relevant to an understanding of what changes can be made in ontogeny, and to link these into certain processes involved in the emergence of leaders in society.

Paul Leyhausen, in his study of the predatory behaviour of cats, has discovered that there are two parts to the performance of catching and killing prey, and that predatory behaviour takes two forms in the adult. The first is more primitive and mainly dependent on genetically programmed instructions (i.e., it is usually called innate). In this form the cat both catches and attempts to kill with its mouth, simultaneously using its canines to dig into the flesh of its prey, but if kittens are given opportunities to imitate their mother and to exercise their propensities to play with prey, they learn a much more sophisticated method which is compounded out of a number of separate parts of behaviour, and which can become integrated into the second type of predatory behaviour largely by imitation and practice. This consists of transferring the act of capture from the jaws to the paws, then throwing the prey, if it small enough, into the air to disorientate it, and this then enables the cat to pounce and kill by biting its neck.

This provides us with the first example of two mutually exclusive alternative types of behaviour being possible in the adult as a result of different experiences during ontogeny.

A second example which shows us how preoccupation with one type of behaviour seems to exclude the development of another faculty in adult life is provided by Neils Bolwig, who kept a young chacma baboon in his family. (You should first realize that baboons brought up in the wild and then caged in captivity have been found inferior to chimpanzees in problem-solving performance (Chance 1960.))

Bolwig discovered that a chacma baboon was capable of solving problems of the same complexity as had been shown possible for captive wild chimpanzees by Kohler in his studies of problem-solving. We are not exactly clear what are the reasons for this, but we know that a great deal of the life of a baboon is spent in jockeying for position in the rank-ordered social relationships which dominate so much of its life, and it may be that this preoccupation excludes practice in problem-solving manipulations. It seems clear, however, that the condition created in baboon society gives no opportunity for the problem-solving faculty to develop. Whatever the reason, this example demonstrates quite clearly that features in the total constellation of a social animal's environment may predispose it to neglect the development of faculties which it otherwise would be able to demonstrate.

It is clearly important that biologists find out what are the alternatives available to any particular species of animal, and perhaps thereby to begin also to aquire insight into the structure of modalities which we inherit from our animal ancestors and some of the likely impediments to changing our behaviour which may be present in us or our ways of life. This is the basis for any discussion of those types of alternatives which are in effect possible for us.

The foregoing evidence has shown that there are well-documented instances in the behaviour of animals which demonstrate that mutually exclusive types of behaviour can develop in the adult. Is there any evidence that such mutually exclusive modalities of behaviour exist or have been demonstrated in our own behaviour?

Arthur Jensen of the Institute of Human Learning, University of California, has evidence that there are two forms of learning that are in one sense mutually exclusive. The first type (type 1) is an ability for association (measured by digital span and serial rote learning tests). Individuals showing this ability are successful in their social relations with other children on the school playground. The second type of learning (type 2) involves the development of conceptual thought (as measured by the Stanford-Binet, Kuhlman-Anderson and Raven's Coloured Progressive Matrices tests). Type 2 learning is nevertheless dependent on the development of type 1 learning, even though it is poorly developed in those that only show type 1.

In my opinion the important point which is overlooked by Jensen is that associative learning (type 1) is used, and therefore specifically expressed, in social behaviour in which involvement of the individual with others is a feature, whereas the other (type 2) is expressed in the solving of problems which do not involve the individual in social relations with others. In the normal life of a person the expression of these two abilities may be specifically linked to the social and non-social activities respectively and, except in situations designed to give the individual an opportunity to express his abilities in other ways, would not normally be dissociated from these forms of behaviour. This distinction indicates that the opportunity to practise social faculties is distinct from and in some sense excludes the development of a faculty which utilizes the other components of intelligence—a suggestive parallel to the example of social/non-social performances which were mutually exclusive in the instance of Bolwig's baboon.

Western democracies are built on the assumption that leaders voted into power are acclaimed for their ability—yet the lessons of European history and most recently the rise of Hitler in Germany provide ample evidence that in times of stress leadership is usurped by individuals who work their way to the centre of social attention, offering panaceas and ultimately dictating social action (Cohn, 1957). It is not difficult to see, therefore, that at times persons reach the status of leaders by appealing directly to the masses and usurping parliamentary authority by modes of charismatic behaviour—this gives them direct non-institutionalized methods of social control—and is another example of two frequently exclusive modes of behaviour.

Why is this so? Francis Williams claims that such was the incompetence of the leaders of England in the 1930's that some explanation is needed as to how they managed to retain power even inside the institutions of democracy. As an illustration of how the incompetence of the banking world grew out of dependency on a man who had no clear ideas about what he was doing, the following quotations from Chapter 8, page 214, of Francis Williams' book will show. Of Montagu Norman (director of the Bank of England) he writes . . .

"He moved about his world like a conqueror whose every word was wrung dry for its significance."

and yet in reply to Ernest Bevin, who questioned him on behalf of the Macmillan committee on Finance and Industry in 1930–31 Norman gave the following reply . . .

"of course you may complain, Mr. Bevin, of me and of those bankers you have seen, that the evidence they have given comes through their nose and is not sufficiently technical or expert. Of course that may in some measure be true; I plead guilty to it myself to some extent and it is a curious thing, that so many of those who inhabit the City find difficulty in stating the reasons for the faith that is in them."

Since this was a time of continuing crisis it seems at least possible that part of a leader's control at any time is partly dependent on non-institutionalized methods and he suggests that these lay in the social relations between the leader and his immediate associates. If this method of control is dependent on a different modality of behaviour from that through which intelligent control is manifest, as in the examples provided by Bolwig and Jensen, we may perhaps have a clue as to why democratic procedures so clearly tend to be disrupted without the participants being aware of what is happening. It is perhaps because the different types of leaders are operating in different modalities of behaviour.

It is now becoming clear that not only many sub-human primate societies (e.g. gorilla, chimpanzee, macaque and savannah baboon), but also simple human societies, are centripetally organized (Chance and Jolly, 1969; Tiger, 1969). These societies possess as a pivoted structure a rank order of males, and in times of crisis all individuals seek the dominant male, who is thus the centre of the society around which all other individuals organize their behaviour. (Of very great importance is a recent discovery by Reynolds and Luscombe that in chimpanzees, social behaviour is rank-ordered by the display potential of individuals.)

I have shown elsewhere (Chance, 1966) that in a centripetal social group a strong tendency to escape makes most of the individuals seek the whereabouts of the dominant male and clump together by running towards him, but makes low ranking animals leave the group.

In sub-human primates, conflicting social tendencies arise in the individuals seeking positions close to the dominant male because all these tendencies are aroused at the same time, and they are at least partially directed towards the dominant male, but can nevertheless not be satisfied in their relation to him. Conflicts also arise between an individual and others competing for status at the centre. In these circumstances conflicts in an individual's social relations can only be resolved by rapid adjustments to the constantly changing events and by the employment of intelligence, involving familiarization, abstraction and integration as a way of reducing the arousal effects of the repeatedly unfamiliar and unexpected events in this social situation.

Man's intelligence can be used to promote the social status of the individual and to directly relate him at any one moment to his social, political or business companions without himself becoming socially involved with them. There is, however, another way for an individual to promote his own status, and that is if he comes under the influence of the instinctive ability (which is in all of us) to make himself the centre of social attention, and which is probably inherited from an earlier phase of evolution as it is seen clearly in the behaviour of sub-human primates.

We have already pointed out that different behavioural abilities come into operation when a person is socially involved rather than otherwise; I suggest that where this primitive social propensity is allowed practice during ontogeny without encouraging the development of intelligence in a child this promotes essentially charismatic social characteristics in an adult, unaccompanied by a complementary ability (necessary in an advanced civilization) for understanding society and its requirements. Hence one of the things we must try to discover is how to encourage social involvement as a basis for a socially competent intelligence, and to discourage social competence unaccompanied by an awareness of the nature of society, and this will involve a major expansion of effort in the social sciences.

So far this argument has been concerned with individuals in their actions directed towards the centre or organizing focus of the society; now I want to consider some of the ethologically definable pitfalls that make it difficult for the individual to operate intelligently, or even discourage him from taking this type of social initiative.

Apparently social involvement, or an individual's estimate of his performances in ranked social relations, can affect his performance on essentially non-social tasks. Robert R. Sears drew attention to a significant interaction between attention to social ranking and test performances a long time ago. He showed how performance in a series of test situations was powerfully influenced by an individual's feelings of relative social position rather than by his actual ability to perform the given tasks. False information to an individual about his relative performance, *vis-à-vis* other candidates, in the previous test reduces his ability to explore all the information available to him in sub-sequent tests, because the individual, disheartened by his apparent social inferiority, withdraws from further exploration of the possibilities, i.e. he escapes from the test situation, reacting to it as if he were withdrawing from the group. Just as those who escape from and leave the society are no longer in receipt of information essential for the solution of social problems, so they are no longer able to solve other types of problems by failing to remain in touch with them. Such socially withdrawn individuals are also prone to another element of behaviour which disrupts the operation of intelligence. Because there are many other cultural influences "keeping people together", this may influence an individual's relations to others when he is highly escape-motivated and cannot get away. This was given the name of *protean* behaviour by Chance and Russell (see Chance, 1963) and is a built-in erratic component enhancing the possibility of successful escape. The erratic component not only disrupts the co-ordination of movement and its orientation, but also the structure of mood. It is part of the escape system of an animal, and similar features are present in many species of vertebrate, as shown by Driver and Humphries (1966).

I shall now return to the point about our own society with which I started. If intelligence is to be the guiding principle of society, then we should encourage those individuals, who happen by their high escape motivation to be prone to the disruptive influences of protean behaviour, to exercise those social faculties which bring them back into the social fold as a pre-requisite for overcoming their asocial tendencies and developing the necessary foundation for the exercise of their intelligence. What we want to do is to encourage those individuals who are highly escape-motivated to develop their capabilities for intelligence, and this means inspiring them towards positive social achievement, instead of overloading their minds with formal and technical education, producing not only a revulsion against the subjects taught, but also thereby enhancing social withdrawal and other elements of their nature disruptive of intelligent behaviour.

Finally, in conclusion, let us be clear that whereas discussion of ethics carried on by traditional disciplines is concerned with the way in which the patterns of behaviour in a society are passed down from the actual authority (see Foss and Richards, this book), my concern has been to show how, through behaviour studies, we may discover the way to encourage the exercise of intelligent judgment in democrats, whose duty today should be to learn how to use their intelligence to establish competent authority and thereafter to know how to brief their leaders; not just, as at present, to live with, and solve piecemeal, the problems created by authority.

REFERENCES

Bolwig, N. (1963). Observations on the Mental and Manipulative Abilities of a Captive Baboon (*Papio doguera*). *Behaviour*, **22**, 1–2, 24–40.

Chance, M. R. A. (1954). The Suppression of Audiogenic Hyperexcitement by Learning *Peromyscus Maniculatus*. *Br. J. Anim. Behav.* **2**, No. 1, Jan.

Chance, M. R. A. (1960) Kohler's Chimpanzees—How did they perform? *Man*, **179**, 1—6.

Chance, M. R. A. (1963). A Biological Perspective on Convulsions. *Colloques Int. Cent. natn. Rech. scient.* (*Paris*) **12**.

Chance, M. R. A. (1966). Resolution of Conflict in Animals and Man. *In:* "Conflict in Society". Ciba Foundation Symposium. (A. V. S. de Reuck and J. Knight, ed.). Churchill, London, England.

Chance, M. R. A. and Jolly, C. J. (1969). Sub-human Primates and their Social Life. (In prep).

Cohn, N. (1957). "The Pursuit of the Millennium". Mercury Books, London, England.

Driver, P. M. and Humphries, D. A. (1966). Protean Behaviour (Systematic Unpredictability in Interspecific Encounters). Ment. Hlth. Res. Inst., *Prepr. No. 197*. University of Michigan, U.S.A.

Jensen, A. R. (1968). Patterns of Mental Ability and Socioeconomic Status. *Proc. Natn. Acad. Sci.* **60,** 1330–1337.

Leyhausen, P. (1965). Uber die funktion der relativen stimmerunghierarchie (Dargestellt ambiespiel der phylogenetischen und ontogenetischen entwicklung des beutefangs von raubtierem). *Z. Tierpsychol.* Band 22, Heft 4 S, 412–494.

Reynolds, V. and Luscombe, G. (1969). Chimpanzee Rank Order and the Function of Displays. (In press).

Sears, R. R. (1944). Success and Failure; a Study in Mobility. *In:* "Studies in Personality", (G. McNemar and M. M. James, ed.).

Tiger, L. (1969). "Men in Groups". Thomas Nelson, London, England.

Waddington (1960). "The Ethical Animal". Allen and Unwin, London, England.

Williams, F. (1965). "A Pattern of Rulers". Longmans, London, England.

The Development of Moral Attitudes and Behaviour

B. M. FOSS

Department of Psychology, Bedford College, Regent's Park, London, England

INTRODUCTION

Attitudes are usually studied by considering what people say rather than do. The relation between saying and doing is not high. For instance, there may be a discrepancy between one's expressed attitude to a person of another race and how one actually behaves to such a person (LaPiere, 1934). It is not known whether this lack of correlation increases or decreases with age. In one study (Belbin, 1956) which had nothing to do with morals, but which was concerned with learning to follow rules, the investigator found that both children and adults show a general lack of relation between the verbal recall of rules or instructions and the putting of them into practice. For such reasons, and also because the development of moral attitudes and behaviour may depend on different mechanisms, the two will be considered separately. As it happens, the empirical studies tend to be based on different samples— attitudes have been studied mainly in normal children and adults, whereas "moral behaviour" has been studied in its relative absence in those who have fallen foul of the law, or of their teachers, or who have certain so-called behaviour disorders.

THE DEVELOPMENT OF MORAL ATTITUDES AND JUDGEMENTS

The development of moral attitudes and judgements depends at least on the following four points.

An appropriate level of cognitive development.

Being exposed to appropriate attitudes and judgements expressed for instance by parents and peers.

What can be called the "psychological distance" of the events and participants which are being judged.

The conditions under which the attitude or judgement is being elicited, especially who is asking the questions.

15

COGNITIVE DEVELOPMENT

The dependence on cognitive development is illustrated by Piaget's experiments (substantially repeated many times) in which a child is required to judge the relative wickedness of various kinds of behaviour (Flavell, 1963, pp. 290–7). A general finding is that a child under eight years old (roughly) does not distinguish between an intentional wrong-doing and one that is a mere accident. For instance, he will judge that the intentional breaking of an object worth so much is not as wicked as the accidental breaking of something worth ten times as much. Motives are not considered and *punishment should be inevitable*. "Mature" judgments may be expected at say 10, and adequate thinking processes to produce them develop in most children. However, it may be noted that an adult who is otherwise reasonable may show punitive behaviour towards another adult even though the other's actions are known to be unintentional.

EXPOSURE TO JUDGEMENTS

The actual judgements made, whatever their developmental status, will depend on the views which a child hears being expressed around him. It has been shown (Bandura and Walters, 1963) that, even though a child has advanced to basing his judgements on whether or not an action was intended, he may nevertheless revert to expressing the less mature judgement if he hears adults expressing that judgement. Conversely, a child may express maturer judgements earlier by being exposed to them earlier. Whom does a child copy in adopting moral judgements? The answer has to be vague since much of the evidence is not rigorously obtained; but early judgements appear to be copied from other members of the family, and misapplied, since the principles have not been understood. Before adolescence there is some evidence that attitudes are adopted increasingly from outside the family, sometimes from fictional and mass media characters, and, of course, from peer groups; indeed from any group with which the child identifies himself, though he may not be a member of it. The concept of identification, deriving from Freud, may be little more than a restatement that the child is adopting the attitudes of a certain group. However, some theories of identification do make predictions, for instance that the child may "identify with the aggressor"; or identify with the status person who dispenses rewards and punishments. Many psychologists would use this concept of identification to explain the copying of moral judgements as well as attitudes.

"PSYCHOLOGICAL DISTANCE"

If a child is asked to judge a person's behaviour, the direction and strength of his judgement depends on what can be called the "psychological distance" of the person being judged. The child's judgment will tend to be neutral if the person being judged is distant geographically or temporally (Rackham, 1966). The child will be the more involved the easier it is for him to identify himself with the person being judged, or the victims, if any. The same factor may affect adults' judgements. If the judge does identify himself with the person being judged, then the sign and strength of his judgement—whether it is punitive, or approving, or permissive—is said to depend on whether the judge exhibits that behaviour himself, and, if so, whether or not he has insight into his own motives.

CONDITIONS

The expression of moral judgements and attitudes depends on the social context. Most people will modify their attitudes depending on who is listening.

THE DEVELOPMENT OF MORAL BEHAVIOUR

Moral behaviour is concerned with the pursuit of worthy goals as well as the avoidance of wrong-doing; however, here we will confine ourselves mainly to avoidance. Moral behaviour is not a category used by psychologists. What is considered moral will depend on the social context—on the group, the religion, the professional ethic, the culture. But in all cases, for the individual, behaving morally involves following rules laid down by someone else. Psychologically then, the development of moral behaviour is a special case of learning to follow rules. Except that "rules" implies that the prescriptions have been codified, or at least verbalized, which is often not the case; so that one must also consider some kinds of moral development as being special cases of becoming conformist.

In the development of an ability to obey verbalized codified rules, Piaget showed that the "immature" judgement (up to, say, eight years) regards rules as strict and almost mythically god-given, and the breaking of them requires punishment, whereas the mature judgement goes with seeing that rules can be changed by mutual consent and are intended to be socially beneficial. Paradoxically, an ability to abide by rules went with seeing that they could be changed. Piaget implies that the authoritarian view of rules is derived from parent-figures and the more mature view comes from experience with peers. This is an attractive theory for which so far there is little evidence.

In learning to follow verbalized rules, the learner has to translate from words to concepts of actions and then to actions, or suppression of actions. It is necessary for the child to have learned the rules, to remember them, to be able to decode them, to have the necessary concepts to be able to put them into action, and to have the motivation necessary to put them into action. It is possible that failure in memory, coding ability or concept formation may sometimes be responsible for failure to behave morally. However, lack of motivation, or competing motivation, is more likely to be the cause.

Here the problem reduces to the more general case of conformity to the particular group norms which define morality.

What processes are involved in learning to conform? Different theorists give different answers. Theories deriving from Freud have put emphasis on modelling or imitation of two kinds—anaclitic identification, which involves modelling oneself on a loved person, and which gives rise to a person's "ego ideal" and desires to do good works; and "identification with the aggressor" which involves the internalization of punishment and the development of conscience. For this kind of theory, the evidence is rather strong that an affectional bond is important for moral development. On the other hand, theories deriving from "learning" theories emphasize the effects of rewards and punishments, and the development of anxiety as a result of conditioning. These theories fit much of the evidence rather well, but are not altogether very satisfactory in explaining the importance of a strong affectional bond.

My own view is that all three mechanisms are involved—rewarding, punishing and imitating. Some of the reinforcements for conformity are obvious, varying from edible or spendable rewards given by parents to prizes and other forms of accolade given by groups and societies to individuals who exemplify what the group or society stands for. However, some rewards are much more subtle. People get pleasure from belonging to a group with common tastes, habits, jargon, beliefs, values. There is an especial pleasure in being physically in a group all admiring one person, or a performance, or a thing, or having a common cause or common activity—or all *disliking* the same person, etc. (It is difficult to reduce this phenomenon to a workable terminology of observables, and psychologists have been successful in dealing with it only at a descriptive level, or by using concepts like identification. It is possible to see that there may be useful functions involved in imitation and conformity, but not so easy to see how pleasurable feelings may result.)

Perhaps the avoidance of punishment, or learning from punishment, is even more potent in producing conformity. Lack of conformity leads to lack of belonging and loneliness, which is punishing. No one has done any counting but it is likely that avoidance of loneliness is a major reason for conforming to some group or other. Other forms of punishment vary from smacking to being laughed at, raised eyebrows, stony silences, hair-shaving and more generally, being made to feel ashamed.

It is possible that the exact way of presenting rewards or punishment may be important. In experiments on puppies, the investigators (Solomon *et al.*, 1968) attempted to train the animals not to eat certain food by cuffing them with a folded newspaper. They were later tested alone with the food, to see if they had developed "consciences". Some puppies had been punished as they were approaching the food, others were punished when they had already eaten some. The first treatment led to a longer avoidance of eating and an apparent development of conscience. The second treatment did not prevent eating, but led to what looked like guilty behaviour after eating. There are related results obtained from experiments with children (Aronfreed and Reber, 1965.)

Some behaviour, for instance exaggeration, may be permitted under some circumstances but not under others. One would expect from other animal work that it would be important for the child that situations where certain behaviour is permitted should be made easily distinguishable from situations where it is forbidden.

The third process is imitation, or copying. This may or may not be reducible to classical conditioning, or to the effects of reward and punishment. For present purposes it will be regarded as a process in its own right, or rather several processes, since there are many kinds of imitation. A child may develop morally, or at least, may come to conform to certain norms, not as a result of any obvious rewards and punishments but through modelling himself on others. (Anyone who has watched a girl of three copying her mother's housekeeping behaviour will agree that to explain the copying in terms of operant or classical conditioning, or combinations of them, is tortuous.) Older children may seek to join groups that have the same interests and ways of behaving that they do, but once in the group, they will imitate further and come to conform—in taste in clothes, hair, make-up, food, drink, entertainment, language, beliefs, values, dislikes and morals. Some prediction is possible, since all of a child's (or adult's) tastes and values, etc., are not likely to change together. Predicting what group a child will see himself as joining, or more simply, predicting how a child will come to see himself, is difficult more because of the number of variables involved rather than through ignorance of the processes. However, some predictions can be made regarding the copying of individual bits of behaviour.

No one ends up as completely conformist, since the various group pressures are balanced by individual drives, for instance in "dominance fighting", status seeking, the need to be different and to be best at something. This jockeying for position can go on within a group or between groups. Once a person has identified with a group, the status of that group will become his own status. Just as an individual may get status in his own group by being the most delinquent, so the group as a whole may be the most delinquent. My impression is that these two kinds of seeking to be different are inversely related; so that, if one is a member of a "way out" group, then one is highly conformist *within* that group.

Although social approval and disapproval continue to influence people to varying extents throughout their lives, nevertheless a person's avoidance of non-moral behaviour is also partly dependent on *a conscience, an internal control* which would operate even if *one knew that there was no chance whatsoever of being found out*. There are several theories to explain how conscience develops, and there is also some empirical evidence on the factors involved. The experiments with puppies were elaborated (Freedman, 1965) so as to demonstrate that a puppy's resistance to temptation depended on its early upbringing. They were most resistant if their upbringing was affectionate but involved correction, and least resistant if it was either punitive or permissive. Comparisons of the families of delinquent and non-delin-quent boys (Bandura and Walters, 1959; Glueck and Glueck, 1950) show fairly reliably that the non-delinquent is more likely to have an affectionate tie with his parents but that also the parents have imposed some discipline, more usually by means of psychological deterrence, such as threatened withdrawal of affection, rather than aggressive verbal or physical punishment. Also, the parents use more explanation; presumably the child is more likely to appreciate underlying principles, if they exist.

In attempting to take a biological approach to these questions, it would seem that, for animals that live in groups, as man does, the evolutionary value of behaviour shifts from that which is important for individual survival to that which is important for group survival. It is to be expected that such survival will depend largely on the evolution of the structures of the groups themselves, but it is also possible that new individual characteristics may come to be selected. For instance, it is conceivable that a change which resulted in an increase in suggestibility (of the kind which is related to an individual's proneness to be led) might result in increased viability for the group, even though the increased suggestibility might have mildly noxious consequences for the individual. However, whereas in lower animals one would expect "altruistic" forms of behaviour to depend on instinctive mechanisms, in man one would expect them to depend largely on learning. In many cases the mores imposed on the individual result in conflict. People may have more aggressiveness and sexuality than society expects to be displayed, and individuals must achieve some compromise between what they want and what is expected. Whether or not a person comes to behave morally, and the consequences for him of doing so, will therefore be related to the individual's style in dealing with conflict. Both highly moral and highly non-moral behaviour may be associated with neurosis.

Is there any evidence for the existence of a moral type of person? Some experimental studies of lying and cheating (Hartshorne and May, 1928) show that there are only low positive correlations between scores of dishonesty in different situations, suggesting that these (rather minor) forms of immorality may be specific to situations. However, as already mentioned, there is evidence that delinquents do show some characteristic differences.

There have been several attempts to develop typologies related to morality, but it is unlikely that there are clear cut all-or-none cases. There are probably the following underlying dimensions:

(i) the internalized standards of conduct may be strong or weak

(ii) those standards may be conventional or deviant

(iii) the person's impulses may be strong or weak

(iv) they may be normal or deviant

(v) the conflict between impulses and standards may have been resolved in various ways

(vi) there may be a physical or functional abnormality

(vii) there may be an important genetic component involved in an inability to behave morally

(viii) immediate environmental factors, including social and economic factors, may be particularly strong ("everybody's doing it").

In conclusion, one can say that there are a very large number of factors determining whether or not a child develops moral behaviour.

For instance, one can catalogue a score of possible causes of failure to learn from the effects of reinforcement. One would be highly suspicious of explanations in terms of any one theory.

REFERENCES

Aronfreed, J. and Reber, A. (1965). Internalised Behavioral Suppression and the Timing of Social Punishment. *J. Personality Soc. Psychol.* **1.**

Bandura, A. and Walters, R. H. (1959). "Adolescent Aggression". Ronald, New York, U.S.A.

Bandura, A. and Walters, R. H. (1963). "Social Learning and Personality Development". Holt, Rinehart & Winston. New York, U.S.A.

Belbin, E. (1956). The Effects of Propaganda on Recall, Recognition and Behaviour. *Br. J. Psychol.* **47,** 163–174; 259–270.

Flavell, J. H. (1963). "The Developmental Psychology of Jean Piaget". Van Nostrand, Princeton, U.S.A.

Freedman, D. G. (1965). Some Effects of Early Rearing on Later Obedience in Dogs. *Nordisk Veterinoermedicin,* **17,** 3–7.

Glueck, S. and Glueck, E. (1950). "Unraveling Juvenile Delinquency". Commonwealth Fund, New York, U.S.A.

Hartshorne, H. and May. M. A. (1928). "Studies in the Nature of Character". Vol. I. Macmillan, New York, U.S.A.

LaPiere, R. T. (1934). Attitudes vs. Actions. *Social Forces,* **13,** 230–7.

Rackham, N. (1966). "An Investigation of Psychological Distance as a Factor Influencing Children's Moral Judgments". Unpublished dissertation, University of Sheffield, England.

Solomon, R. L., Turner, L. H. and Lessac, M. S. (1968). Some Effects of Delay of Punishment on Resistance to Temptation in Dogs. *J. Personality Soc. Psychol.* **8,** No. 3, 233–38.

Characteristics of Ethical Systems in
Primitive Human Society

AUDREY I. RICHARDS

University of Cambridge, Cambridge, England

INTRODUCTION

I suspect that anthropologists were asked to contribute to this
Symposium because the type of societies they commonly study are
popularly considered to occupy a sort of halfway stage between animal
communities and those of modern industrial society.

Like the animal societies, these primitive human communities are
small in size. I suppose that it is impossible to give a figure for the
average size of colonies of the lower primates or of packs or herds of
other mammals, but the societies that have been studied by anthropologists are often very small when compared with our own. Along
the New Guinea coast, for example, there are groups of 800—1000
people claiming a separate identity, speaking a common language and
exhibiting a common culture. The Trobriand islanders, familiar to the
psychoanalyst and the sociologist through the work of Malinowski,
numbered not more than 1300 when he visited them in 1914; and
120—200,000 would be an average figure for the Bantu tribes of east
and central Africa. The face-to-face communities—the homestead,
settlement, or village—may range from 5—6 families to a village of
150—200 individuals. As in the case of animal societies, these are
groups based on biological ties (using this term very loosely), i.e. they
are groups composed of a few individuals and their respective descend-
ants. In human communities these groups include members of three
or four generations; in animal communities the depth of the group
based on common descent is presumably less, owing to the shorter
span of life of the individuals concerned.

As in many animal societies, some kind of authority is accepted
in most primitive human communities, a ranking order or the
acknowledgement of a leader or a hierarchy of leaders. In both types
of society privileges over food or other scarce resources are claimed by
some members of the group and not others. There are also accepted

23

rights over territory—whether it be used in a human society for cultivation or merely for hunting and fishing.

Here, however, the similarities probably end. Primitive societies, of course, share with those of the modern industrial world the fact that their behaviour is governed by a culture transmitted from generation to generation in the form of language, knowledge, rules, systems of social grouping, beliefs and material objects. The members of such communities feel a sense of common identity based on a transmitted memory of the past; they are governed by a system of values and they have a power of conceptualizing social relationships. Although the small local communities characteristic of primitive societies cease to consist of simple biological families, elaborate kinship terminologies make it possible for the individuals concerned to regard themselves as though they were members of such families. This is done by extending terms primarily used for biological relationships (such as parent to child, child to parent, or sibling to sibling) to a number of persons of agnatic or collateral descent who may have very few genes in common when the linguistic extension is at its widest.

So also are the hierarchies of authority positions, which appear to resemble the ranking orders of animal societies, distinguished by linguistic usage and traditional status obligations which are passed from generation to generation, and learned by members of those generations. They are not established afresh on the basis of the relative physical strength of the individuals in each small local group.

The Anthropological Approach to the Study of Ethics

Anthropologists are bound to study the ethical codes of the people they are observing. They find this necessary because the nature of their material, as well as their training, encourages them to view the cultures they are studying as systems—systems of social relationships, of organized activities, or of ideas and beliefs. Ethical codes and values are an essential part of these systems in the sense that the institutions of the society would not work without them.

Anthropologists have perhaps a particular approach to the study of ethics. It is an outlook dictated by their traditional interests and also by the type of data they are able to use. They have, for the most part, described ethical principles in terms of the obligations accepted by the members of a community rather than as abstract virtues such as courage, loyalty to the group, industry, or a sense of justice. This is partly because the communities they commonly study come under the category of "closed societies" rather than open—categories to which

Professor Mitchell refers (page 37). It is the practical experience of anthropologists that the peoples among whom they are working tend to praise a man for deeds such as caring for his dead sister's children; or looking after his brother's widow; or for carrying out the commands of a chief faithfully. They rarely describe this behaviour as altruism or loyalty.

However, the outlook of anthropologists is also explained by their primary interest, which is the study of the functioning of particular societies. This is especially true if it is a community not previously described. For this reason anthropologists tend to consider codes of behaviour in so far as they help or hinder the conduct of the major activities of the tribe, e.g. its organization for war; its trading systems; or its methods of settling disputes.

Anthropologists are also much influenced by the type of observations which they have to make in the field, and their approach is evidently a highly empirical one. A behaviourist attitude is forced on them by the nature of their material. Anthropologists of the classical period, i.e. those who were making field studies in the thirties, had to make their observations in pre-literate societies—although there are a few completely illiterate peoples at the present day. Fieldworkers therefore had available no *corpus* of the ethical rules of the community in print; no tables of stone; no legal codes; no church liturgies or philosophical works. For this reason they had to rely on a series of oral statements or direct personal observations. Oral statements may be made on formal occasions such as the instructions given to those assuming new roles—e.g. to a man assuming a new office who may be instructed to be wise, merciful, fierce or just, according to the ideals of his community. The duties of husband and wife are announced in most marriage ceremonies including those of the Christian church. Judges in primitive societies as well as those in our own legal courts make formal pronouncements of values when giving judgement. They may say, for example, "this idle and pleasure-loving woman", the definition of idleness and a culpable enjoyment of pleasure being assumed to be that current in the community at the time. In primitive societies, the words of the lamentations at a funeral may also make formal pronouncements as to the virtues that the dead have exercised or are supposed to have exercised.

It may be difficult to imagine ourselves constructing a picture of, for example, Christian ethics in our own society, entirely on the basis of formal pronouncements so collected, but this is just what anthropologists have to try to do.

Anthropological fieldworkers also use informal comments heard, or overheard in the course of village life; ejaculations, shouts, or abuse uttered in the course of quarrels, or the taunts and laughter aroused by non-conformity. Such spontaneous comments are obviously most frequently made in the case of broken rules and the community's reactions to such behaviour. Hoebbels calls the deductions made from such incidents "the trouble case method". Men and women confronted by a new ethic, such as a Christian code taught in a pagan society, may also be surprised into making revealing comments on their own values.

Anthropologists also try to deduce some of the ethical rules that are obeyed almost unconsciously by the people concerned, even if they are not expressed in words. The statistical analysis of case-histories, say of marriage or divorce, may reveal uniformities indicating the acceptance of a rule of which the people seem unaware until they are specifically challenged. The figures may also, of course, show the extent to which they are deviating from the rules they express in formal terms. Professor Foss reminds us (page 15) of the difference between what people say and what they do, and such a discrepancy is inevitable, since most ethical rules are framed in order to persuade men and women to do things they do not want to do, or to abstain from doing things which they would very much like to do. The relation between the pronounced norm and the statistical norm is now considered a necessary part of the highly empirical type of study of ethics which anthropologists try to conduct. Recent attempts to concentrate on the cognitive systems of primitive peoples and their use of symbols in ritual and myth have proved rewarding and fascinating, but symbolism is not a very useful guide to the ethical system of a particular people.

AREAS OF ETHICAL CONTROL

Starting from this severely empirical basis I think I can best make a contribution to this book by describing the areas of behaviour which tend to be governed by rules and to be enforced by sanctions, whether positive or negative. Leach has recently denied the existence of any universal rules of morality except, perhaps, those forbidding mother-son incest. "Codes are arbitrary", he says, "and change from place to place". It is true, of course, that morals and values vary from culture to culture, but I think that the areas of behaviour governed by such rules vary very much less, if at all. We may be brought up in societies in which it is thought essential for a man to have only one wife; or in which four is the limit permitted; or among people who consider it admirable to have as many wives as possible. But a society has not yet been discovered without some rule governing the right to produce children and the duty of rearing them.

What, then, are the areas of behaviour which are characteristically subject to rule in primitive as distinct from modern society?

Sex and Parenthood

I think first and foremost comes the proliferation of rules of conduct centring round the control of mating and the production of children—regulations, taboos and moral principles which far exceed those in our present day society. They include:

(a) *Mating rules and attitudes.* Mating behaviour is certainly patterned in all communities, animal and human. Since individuals of both sexes are involved there must be some recognizable signs of acceptance or refusal between both. But in human society ideals of male and female beauty or mate-worthiness are taught, and largely depend on cultural factors. More than this, in primitive societies the choice of mate in marriage is subject to innumerable prohibitions and injunctions. Sometimes these apply to casual mating but more usually only in the case of mating leading to parenthood and the founding of a family as a social unit. The prohibitions involve the universal taboos on incest between close relatives in the family (parent-child or sibling-sibling), but the rules are commonly extended in primitive societies to a whole generation of men and women in a single line of descent—men and women to whom *ego* extends the "father" or "mother" term; the "brother" or "sister" term in his or her own generation; and the "son" or "daughter" terms in the one below. The breaking of these rules of clan or lineage incest is felt to be morally wrong and liable to divine and human punishment.

In primitive societies it is also common to find positive injunctions to contract special types of marriage as well as prohibitions on a wide range of unions. Endogamy, or the injunction to marry within a clan or village, is quite frequent and special approval of marriages between men and women within one social class is very common indeed. Preferred marriages between cross-cousins, often associated with the inheritance of property or economic exchanges between two groups united by marriage, are also common. Societies of this type are, in fact, divided into marriageable and non-marriageable men and women—a contrast to our own society in which incest within the biological family is virtually the only type of mating which is forbidden.

It is remarkable how easily children come to accept the categories of the marriageable and the non-marriageable. This is chiefly, I think, because they acquire the requisite patterns of behaviour early in life when they are mocked if they make mistakes between their "brothers" and their "cross-cousins". The kinship nomenclature enables them to extend the behaviour proper to a "brother" or a "sister" to the limits of clan.

Human societies prescribe the number of mates possible in marriage, whether the rule is for monogamy for both sexes or for one sex only, as in the different forms of polygyny and polyandry. Extra marital intercourse is also commonly regulated as well as the time in life when marriages may be contracted—after service as a warrior for instance.

It was rather naïvely assumed at the beginning of the century that these mating rules had a useful biological function; that the regulations prevented inbreeding, then thought to be inevitably disastrous. The rules, of course, do not prevent inbreeding. By a preferential cross-cousin marriage a man may produce children by the daughter of his father's sister or of his mother's brother and he is enjoined to do so. Exogamy rules merely prevent him marrying the daughter of his father's brothers or his mother's sister, the children of siblings of the same sex. We now see the mating rules of primitive societies as having almost entirely social functions as, for instance, governing the alliances between two groups, sometimes united by the continuous exchange of women and goods (see the Kriges' description of Lovedu marriage). The rules may govern the orderly passage of property and determine the control of children, so much desired in societies of this type. They avoid or greatly reduce conflicts over mates. Marriage rules form social categories which may be the basis of systems of economic co-operation by which a group of men and their relatives in law are pledged to work in an exchange relation. It would be more valid to say that social values had biological results, e.g. on the fertility of women,* than that these rules were themselves the results of biological needs.

(b) *Parenthood*. In primitive communities the rewards given to those who produce and rear offspring tend to be much greater than in our own. Children are much desired in communities where the infant mortality is high. They are the means of founding a family in a society in which the family is the basic unit of residence, economic and political activities and legal affiliation. In these circumstances the larger the biological family, the larger and more powerful the lineage, the village

---

* F. Lorimer has specifically studied the effects of cultural rules such as postponing the age of mating for women, limiting their choice of mate, preventing the re-marriage of widows, etc. on human fertility (see Lorimer, 1954).

and the clan. In our society parents are constantly warned of the dangers of over-population. They tend to be admired for sexual prowess but rarely for their success as procreators and rearers of children. By contrast the emphasis in primitive societies is on parenthood. Fathers and mothers are given high status and in some cases addressed by the names of their children as a term of respect, that is to say, as "Father of Mary" or "Mother of John"; the barren woman is liable to divorce; the childless man usually has a lower social and political status. Parenthood is associated with good fortune, supernatural favour, immortality and the continuity of the group; fertility magic centres round the nubile girl and the young married couple. Child-birth is associated with taboos specially designed to emphasize the social role of the parents and particularly of the father of the baby.

In spite of this emphasis on procreation it must be stressed that the production of offspring is not regarded as an end in itself—children must be produced for a particular group. They must be born in marriage, the institution which allocates children to particular lines of descent, whether patrilineal or matrilineal, and gives them rights to care, inheritance or succession in that group. They are, in fact, "legitimate" children and the fact is emphasized in most societies of this type by naming or other ceremonies designed to express the group's acceptance of its obligations to the child. This is done to avoid conflict as to the lineage he belongs to. The right to reproduce is, in fact, quite closely determined and in those societies in which premarital intercourse is licensed, then the couples are scolded if they produce children before marriage. For instance, intercourse must be incomplete when girls visit their lovers in the barracks of the unmarried warriors in some East African tribes.

The distinction between the social and the biological father, between the *pater* and the *genitor*, is clearly marked in these societies, with the emphasis always on the former—the social father, who makes the marriage payment for the mother to acquire legitimate rights over the children she bears him. The great emphasis on the social duties of father and mother has led some of my colleagues to deny that the biological ties between mating couples and their offspring in human society have much significance. They point to such wide-spread customs as adoption and the exchange of children between groups to cement unity; to the superior rights of the social to the biological father, and many similar customs.* I cannot go as far as this. One has

---

* Even women can become social fathers in some African societies since a wealthy woman can make a payment for a young girl and secure paternal rights over the children the father bears by lovers. She is even addressed as "father" by these children.

to remember that it is the biological urge to mate which societies
attempt to control (however imperfectly) by a battery of ethical rules
and negative and positive sanctions; that social inducements reinforce
the instinctive parental endowment and persuade fathers and mothers
to perform their prescribed role for many years; and that in primitive
society most social groups are conceived of in the pattern of the
biological family.

(c) *Succour and protection*. Other primates extend the nurturant role
of mother to infant to other members of the community, to the young,
sick or wounded; and there are certainly very strongly sanctioned
rules in primitive societies enforcing succour to the afflicted within
an extended circle of kinsmen, and the sharing of supplies within
the group. It is considered the duty of *ego* to look after his parents;
his siblings—real or classificatory; his sibling's children; his grand-
children, and other categories of kinsmen. Such conduct is admired.
It is also enforced very often by fear of supernatural punishment,
such as the anger of the ancestors, the dread of provoking hostile
public opinion and the forces of reciprocity. "If you do not give me
refuge when elephants have trampled on my gardens, then I shall
certainly turn a deaf ear when you are in the same trouble". Such
mutual help is necessary as a social insurance in societies in which
there is no source of help outside the kinship system, but also, by a
secondary extension, the exchange of services and goods comes to be
undertaken as a symbol of these very kinship ties; to express or maintain them; or to acquire high status by constantly giving and putting
others under an obligation to you. Thus a man may give food to X
because he arrives on the door-step as a starving brother, but he may
also carry baskets of food long distances to relatives in another village
to express respect or to "keep the kinship warm" between himself and
his relatives in-law.

The sharing of food is one of the first lessons in social behaviour
learnt by children in societies of this type. In a Bemba village in
Zambia, in which education was of a most permissive type, the only
thing for which children were punished was for eating food alone.
I have seen half a banana seized from a screaming three-year-old and
divided into squashed morsels between four other children with the
shout, "You bad child! Trying to eat alone!" The same sort of scene
has been described during the Biafran famine of today. It is doubtful
whether sharing, the basis of this particular system of social insurance,
could be maintained without very early inculcation in this way. Is it
instinctive behaviour shared by some, at any rate, of the other
primates? Is it altruism of the highest sort? Is it behaviour based on

the acceptance of reciprocal obligations acknowledged by members of these typically closed societies?

(d) *Other areas of control*. Ethical principles, of course, govern the use and inheritance of property, and particularly of land and major economic resources in all communities yet described. The individual is protected against injury, assault and murder, and he has well-defined duties in the defence of his community against an outside enemy. However, I feel it impossible to cover such a wide field and have confined myself to those areas of control in which there seem to be more similarities between human and animal societies and in which the differences between primitive and advanced societies seem to be quite marked.

If one can generalize about the ethical systems of primitive peoples I think one would have to emphasize (i) the importance given to enlarging and strengthening the face-to-face community, and to extending its links with other communities. I have instanced the value attached to the procreation and care of children, and to the making and keeping of ties with other groups by the continuous exchange of goods and of women; (ii) the great emphasis placed on the avoidance of conflict within the small communities. All rules of conduct reduce conflict since they lead to expected and therefore acceptable conduct. However, I have described the importance attached to marriage rules in primitive society as a means of avoiding confusion about the control and care of children, their affiliation to different descent lines, their inheritance and succession. Property rules and traditional hierarchies of authority similarly avoid sources of conflict and confusion. The importance attached to machinery for arbitrating in local disputes by provision of outside arbitrators has been stressed by many anthropologists. Ceremonies designed to express the resumption of good relations after a local dispute or ritual symbolizing the removal of evil thoughts, malevolence or witchcraft are also common, as is magic for the maintenance of peaceful village life and the absence of quarrels; (iii) the importance of mutual support as the only possible form of social insurance in communities unusually prone to disasters.

These duties are conceived by the people as a series of rights and obligations acknowledged between categories of men and women in societies made "closed", so to speak, by the extension of kinship terms through large sections of the lineage or clan. While the young in our society resent "paternal behaviour", those in primitive communities extend the term "father" to a number of men who are not their fathers at all and so pledge them to father-like behaviour. An ethical system of this kind is probably easier to teach since the duties involved are concrete and they can be inculcated very early in a child's life, but of course it is not an adaptable method of controlling behaviour or applicable to a society in which even local groups are based on so many principles other than kinship and the child becomes a member of so many groups and categories.

REFERENCES

Krige, J. D. and Krige, E. J. (1947). "The Realm of a Rain Queen".

Leach, E. (1967). "A Runaway World". Reith Lectures 1967, p. 49. BBC, London, England.

Leach, E. (1967). "A Runaway World". Reith Lectures 1967, p. 56. BBC, London, England.

Lorimer, F. (ed.). (1954). "Culture and Human Fertility". UNESCO

Discussion

TOWERS: Professor Foss says in his paper, "It would seem that, for animals that live in groups, as man does, the evolutionary value of behaviour shifts from that which is important for individual survival to that which is important for group survival." It seems to me that the idea that individual survival is—or ever was—of paramount importance represents a serious misunderstanding of the nature of the evolutionary process, a process which always operates at the group or species level and not at that of the individual. The notion that individualistic aggression is a major factor in 'the survival of the fittest' led to terrible social consequences in the nineteenth century, from which we are still suffering. Today we recognize that this is not a basic characteristic of sub-human forms. Co-operative, social activity is much more commonly found in 'lower' forms than used to be thought. Species survival is the only kind of survival that is important in the evolutionary process. So, though of course I agree that in man what is of evolutionary value is 'behaviour which is important for group survival', I would question whether there had to be a 'shift' in order for this to come about. The Spenglerian idea that man's evolutionary inheritance was that of a beast of prey is surely not accepted by reputable biologists, despite its reappearance in recent popular books.

EBLING: Men may experience conflict in conforming to rules but they seem at some stage or another to acquire attitudes and beliefs—even ones which are out-of-date and quite irrelevant to current society—with terrifying ease. Is this process the same as other kinds of learning?

FOSS: There are many kinds of learning, which may or may not have something in common at a molecular level. The acquiring of attitudes and beliefs seems to depend partly on 'identifying' with someone, or a group of people, or a cause; and there isn't the same pressure to modify beliefs in the light of evidence as there is to modify behaviour as a result of rewards and punishments. It is possible that 'identifying' may turn out to be a kind of conditioning, though some psychologists would say it is more complicated.

EBLING: I wondered if anything was known of possible neurological mechanisms connected with the acquisition of moral attitudes? Does prefrontal leucotomy, for example, alter ethical feelings?

FOSS: Probably. It can certainly result in behaviour which appears to me much less concerned with 'what people think of me'. This could be due to a lot of things—for instance, a failure to anticipate the consequences of one's actions. In which case the neurological mechanism involved might be related to anticipation rather than 'ethical feelings'.

BUSVINE: It has been pointed out that the survival or decline of a human culture is quite distinct and separate from the proliferation or dwindling of the people who practise it. Characters which favour the growth and survival of the culture may or may not benefit the people who originate it. While a Darwinian type of 'survival of the fittest' cannot apply to cultures in a strict sense, yet something analogous presumably occurs. It is often assumed that rather aggressive and repressive cultures would be expected to flourish. But is this, in fact, so? Possibly the vigorous, aggressive and coercive social systems we have seen in the past few decades contain seeds of weakness. By their repression of more sensitive and liberal individuals (resulting in many of these emigrating) they may deprive the whole society of much intellectual capital.

DE REUCK: Ethical systems—even in the rare cases where they are acted upon by a majority of the population for most of the time—cannot be regarded as necessarily conferring a selective breeding advantage on their practitioners. High moral standards have no survival value for either individual or the species—on the contrary, the brave and altruistic may feel called upon to sacrifice themselves for the rest of the community in time of crisis. Morals are culturally transmitted behavioural traits and, in general, natural selection does not operate on cultural traits. It is not possible to ascribe cultural evolution to a process of natural selection that encourages the persistence of 'good' social customs and eliminates maladaptive ones. The pace of social change is too fast for any such balance to be achieved. Ideas or habits do not persist primarily because their owners have more children, nor are they dropped merely because their owners die. Of course, certain customs, like eating poisonous berries or remaining celibate on religious grounds, would literally die out rapidly if they were widely adopted, but within the broad limits set by man's biological inheritance, specific items in his repertoire of culturally transmitted behaviour do not, individually, have any significant survival value.

Sociologists suggest that what in fact happens is that a process of social selection operates directly on cultural innovations (mutations) depending on their compatibility with the internal organization and processes of the society in which they arise. It is the social system upon which successful innovations confer an adaptive advantage and not the individual man nor the human species, at any rate directly.

Societies are conceived, in systems analysis terms, as abstract systems or networks of roles, collectives, norms and values—interlocking and interacting so that almost every individual trait reinforces and sustains the actions and expectations of others. Societies are homeostatic systems, with feedback loops for information and energy to regulate their operation about some moving equilibrium, like a developing organism. Now the function of an ethical system is to help to maintain the smooth running and internal stability of society; and the biological function of society is to provide a stable social environment for the development of the human animal.

Maladaptive ethical traits thus destroy, not the men who display them, but the social system that harbours them. That is why missionaries, preaching an alien moral code maladapted to the local society, tend to undermine the whole cultural background of their converts. But it would be a mistake to suppose that natural selection or Darwinian adaptation will give us a clue to selecting the 'best' ethical system.

FRASER DARLING: I would suggest that an ethical attitude is a normal development of human sociality. As soon as two people live together an acceptable behaviour of harmonious living must be reached, which involves restraint and mutual service. When a man and woman find themselves caring for a child, cooperative ethical behaviour is almost inevitable—unless it isn't and then natural selection exerts its own answer. I would also suggest that good manners are natural in primitive human societies and are conducive to the development of ethical attitudes. A Highlander once said to me, "Had we not developed good manners we should not have survived as people." Again, I remember walking alone, thankfully, five miles ahead of a punctured Land Rover, in a remote part of the Darfur province of the Sudan, when a black Arab on a thin horse, a woman riding a bull and another man walking with a laden camel came by. Only the black Arab stopped, sidled towards me with elaborate dressage steps of his horse, and in sign language expressed concern for my safety—no food, no cover, just walking, and it was near dusk. With less fluent mime I explained my situation and expectation of being picked up. We bowed to each other as men of good will, he a man of a tribe given to compulsive violence and I just a Wandering Willie. Surely his concern was the ethical attitude engendered by a harsh environment, concern for survival of another.

BROUGHTON: Professor Chance has warned us of the need for close study of the structure of animal behaviour before attempting applications to human affairs. Several speakers have interpreted one of the bases of ethics as conformism acquired, during development, by learning—a cultural trait, culturally transmitted. Perhaps, in this assumption of learning, we are falling into the pit of anthropomorphism Dr. Fraser Darling warned us against.

A few years ago some of my experimental grasshoppers, animals surely with little real learning ability, showed a surprising degree of temporary conformism. An individual of one species, normally singing disyllabically, when placed a few feet from another species producing unitary sounds, quickly commuted his song to one consisting very preponderantly of monosyllables. This same species, in the presence of a highly polysyllabic species, commuted its song to long and only slightly irregular polysyllabic runs, which endured as long as the opposite number was singing, or a little longer.

Other experiments in the series could be interpreted in terms of simple neurophysiological processes of excitation, inhibition or feedback disruption notions currently being checked in my team. But this apparent numerical matching, of which one or two, less extreme, other examples occur in the literature, hardly could be. The seeming attempt to conform to an alien song pattern, in a group considered to be much more instinct-driven than mammals, must warn us that conformism in the latter and in ourselves may not be primarily based on learning, and may have roots deep in instinctive behaviour. There could be a real 'instinct to conform', based on the selective disadvantage, even at primitive levels, of failing to produce the releasers for tolerance by the group.

The Historical Approach to Ethics, especially those of Christianity

BASIL MITCHELL

Oriel College, Oxford, England

In a chapter entitled 'The Animal with a Conscience' Konrad Lorenz writes, "For a wild animal in its natural state, there is no conflict between natural inclinations and what it 'ought' to do, and this is the paradise which man has lost. The fruits of man's higher mental capacities are his cultural development, and above all, the power of speech and of conceptual thought, and the accumulation and traditional passing on of common knowledge. All this has resulted in man's historical evolution at a rate which is many hundreds of times more rapid than the purely organic genealogical development of all other living beings."

If Lorenz is right—and surely he is—there is no such thing as ethics in the animal world. Yet there are patterns of behaviour which resemble human moral conduct to such an extent as to tempt us to talk about the ethical, or at any rate the "ethical", behaviour of animals. Thus Jonathan Bennett tells us in his book on Rationality that "ants of some species, when on the march in their tens of thousands, will cope with a fire which lies in their path by marching straight into it, the bodies of the first few thousand smothering the fire and the rest marching straight on over." Are the ants brave? Bennett says, "The behaviour of those in front looks like bravery in much the same way as apian dances look like symbolism; yet no-one thinks that ants are either brave or cowardly." He suggests a resolution of the difficulty as follows, "The force of the claim that the dances of the . . . honey-bees 'look symbolic' is just that it looks as though the only reason that bees could have for dancing as they do is to inform one another of the whereabouts of food; and this can be sensibly asserted by someone who does not know whether bees have any reasons for any of their behaviour, or who knows that they do not have reasons for any of their behaviour. Similarly, even if we are confident that ants ought not to be said to have reasons for anything they do, we are entitled to say that if the concepts of 'reason' or 'motive' could be brought to bear upon the behaviour of the ants which march straight into the fire, they would have to be applied in such a way as to justify describing that behaviour as brave, self-sacrificing, etc."

The ants are an interesting case, because we really do have no doubts of the sort we might conceivably have with some of the higher mammals about the impossibility of actually ascribing bravery to them, in spite of the fact that their behaviour in sacrificing their lives in such a way as to preserve the lives of their fellows is exemplary. This requires some explanation. There is, after all, a strong positive analogy with human bravery; hence the appropriateness of this description of what they do. Moreover, the fact that we regard bravery as a moral virtue is obviously not unrelated to our recognition that conduct of this sort tends to the preservation of the group. Whether or not *all* moral virtue has this sort of relation to survival, bravery certainly has.

Why then are we so clear that the ants are *not* brave? There are a number of reasons: (i) while *we* are able to describe their behaviour as "preserving the lives of their fellows at the cost of their own", they are not. They do not even think of their behaviour as "marching straight on into the fire", because they do not think of it at all. Hence it is not an *action* calling for moral assessment of any kind; (ii) *a fortiori* they have no *reasons* for what they do. We can recognize that their behaviour tends to the preservation of the species and has been perpetuated by natural selection, and we can express this in a convenient short-hand by saying that they march on *because* their doing so will help preserve the rest, but this is not to ascribe reasons to them; (iii) there is no conflict (to repeat Lorenz's words) between their natural inclinations and what they "ought" to do. They do not have to overcome fear.

These are valid reasons, but to some they may not seem particularly important in comparison with the following considerations: (i) the behaviour of the ants readily lends itself to description in the same terms as human actions; (ii) it performs a similar function in the preservation of the community against danger as bravery in human beings; (iii) bravery in human beings would not be possible unless men had a natural tendency to aggressive behaviour, or necessary unless men were vulnerable to dangers of the same sort as beset animals. These considerations may tempt us to the view that essentially the "ethical" behaviour of animals and morality in men are identical, or at any rate that they represent alternative ways of achieving an identical end.

Such a view may claim some support from the kind of functional analysis by which social anthropologists seek to explain features of primitive societies (and sometimes of more advanced societies). Thus an explanation may be given of the institution of feuding in terms of the contribution it makes to the stability of a certain form of social organization, whether or not those who engage in the feuds have this as part of their conscious intention or, indeed, even if they have purposes of quite another kind. It is possible to give similar functional accounts of the elements of the moral code of a particular society; and some of these elements—and bravery is a plausible case—may be such that their recognition as part of the code is a necessary condition of the survival of any society whatever. To the extent that interest is concentrated on the "objective" function of courageous behaviour in preserving society, "subjective" factors like the "reasons" and "motives", which Bennett emphasizes as characteristically human, are made to appear somewhat incidental.

Before considering to what extent this kind of analysis is adequate as a complete account of human morality it is perhaps worth noticing that, in spite of similarities of language, such explanations do not always operate with the same concept of survival as that of the animal ethologist and can scarcely make the same use of the idea of natural selection. For to explain a certain institution as tending to promote the survival of a society may mean simply, and usually does mean, not that the society would altogether cease to exist as a society if the institutions were abandoned or radically altered, but that it would become in some significant way a different society, having a different "form of life". It is only if "not surviving" has the force of "ceasing to exist as a society" that the idea of natural selection gets any purchase in this context, i.e. if it can be argued that such and such an institution has remained a feature of a particular society, because otherwise that society would have ceased to exist. The actual utility of this line of argument would appear to be somewhat restricted since, as Dorothy Emmet has pointed out, (a) there does not seem to be much evidence of many societies having died out as distinct from somehow carrying on in a depressed condition, (b) there are so many ways of surviving that the need to survive tells us little of why a society has one institution or one form of an institution rather than others.

However it certainly seems plausible to suggest that bravery at least is a moral virtue which any society must encourage if it is to survive in the straightforward sense of continuing to exist. So it may help if we glance quickly at the development of the concept in the history of our own cultural tradition, starting with the bravery of the Homeric hero, who feels obliged to do what is expected of him as a member of a warrior caste for the sake of his reputation among his peers. Already within a few centuries we find Plato defining courage as "the power of maintaining right and lawful belief concerning what is and what is not to be feared" which he distinguishes from "mere right opinion on these matters such as is not the result of education, but the expression of an animal and slavish nature". Plato's conception of courage is far too intellectualist but it makes it possible to recognize as an example of courage the refusal of Socrates to save his life by repudiating the principles for which he had lived. Courage of this sort requires an independently thought-out philosophy of life in terms of which the individual can reflectively determine "what is and what is not to be feared". This "philosophical" conception of courage was extremely influential in antiquity and, in one form, is eloquently expressed by Cicero, "Reason further contains a noble glorious element, fitted for ruling rather than obeying in such a way as to look on our mortal lot as trivial and easily endurable". Aristotle distinguishes this sort of courage, that of the man who has a reasoned conception of what is worth dying for, from that of the citizen soldier whose motive is the rewards and penalties of society. It was courage so understood which was taken over by Christian writers as one of the cardinal virtues. It is easy to see how it could be developed so as to include the courage of the martyr, though its character might vary according to what precisely it was that the individual saw himself as standing for. At this stage it becomes inevitably more difficult to tell simply by observation of what a man does whether he is exhibiting courage or not. The courage of the man who does not retaliate under extreme provocation is superficially indistinguishable from the inertia of the man who lacks the spirit to resist. Gethsemane would be unintelligible to the Homeric hero.

There seem to be two developments here of permanent significance. One is the rise of critical and creative judgement on the part of the individual. The other is the shift from what Bergson called the "closed" to the "open" society. Socrates and Jesus do not simply internalize the moral codes of their own society; they criticize them in the name of an ideal society. There is some controversy as to the stages by which these developments took place but they both culminated in Christianity. Thus we now take for granted the possibility of a certain sort of altruistic courage, which has been a rare and comparatively recent phenomenon in human history. Vincent Cronin in his biography of Matthew Ricci records the astonishment of the Chinese when Jesuit missionaries dived overboard to rescue some men from drowning. It was, from their point of view, foolhardy. The action had point only if other human beings were thought of as having a unique value, no matter whether they were related to one or how one rated them according to the accepted standards of human worth. The point is well made by Lorenz, "Men can behave very decently indeed in tight spots, provided they are of a kind that occurred often enough in the palaeolithic period to produce phylogenetically adapted social norms that deal with the situation. Loving your neighbour like yourself and risking your life in trying to save him is a matter of course, if he is your best friend and has saved your life a number of times; you do it without even thinking. The situation is entirely different if the man for whose life you are expected to risk your own, or for whom you are supposed to make other sacrifices, is an anonymous contemporary on whom you have never set eyes."

So, as Dorothy Emmet says, " 'open' morality can go beyond, without superseding, the social morality based on expectations as to how people will behave in a recognized system of rights and obligations because it springs from a more disinterested love of man for man. This may show itself either in an enlargement of compassionate imagination, which may make people sensitive to wider ranges of duties beyond those of their 'in-group', or it may show itself in the self-forgetful moral heroism with which they may perform a service to a member of their in-group without thought of return."

What I have very briefly sketched is a historical development owing much to the insight of particular individuals. The communication of fresh moral insight takes place by teaching and example and changes in moral outlook thus communicated have altered the form of entire societies. The rise of the "open" society has brought with it greater opportunities for the individual to make an independent contribution to ethics. Hence insofar as an existing institution or element in a moral code can be explained in terms of the contribution it makes to the survival of a particular form of life, it still stands in need of justification in at least two respects; we need to ask, (a) whether the end could be achieved in a more efficient or a more desirable manner, (b) whether the form of life itself ought to be changed in certain ways. The point has been well put by Professor S. F. Nadel ". . . In analysing any society we cannot but assess its capacity to achieve stability and continuity, to function smoothly and in an integrated fashion, and on this basis evaluate its adequacy . . ." But " . . . a society may achieve its stability or permanence only by the rigid exercise of force, causing deprivation and frustration on a wide scale. In a society which glorifies war or individual rivalry for rank or wealth, the gratifications undoubtedly derived from such an ethos of power and achievement will go together with physical suffering and severe psychological strains. Frustrations and strains may in turn have to be relieved by the catharsis of licensed aggression, say, against witches, scapegoats or 'other enemies of the people'. And only too often do the gratifications of one section of society mean the unfulfilled desires of another". ". . . whether social stability and national glory achieved at the cost of human suffering are worth the price, whether relief from tension through hunting down scapegoats represents a 'good' adjustment to existing conditions, these and similar questions are answerable apparently only in terms of private convictions—about war and peace, individual dignity, or human happiness". As Lorenz emphasizes, we often do not understand the ways in which the various features of our society contribute to our total form of life and both biology and social anthropology can extend our knowledge and so increase our control. But in the end it is what Lorenz calls "responsible morality" which has to decide, among the innumerable possible ways, how we are to live; "Therefore man is forced to test, with the help of conscious thought, every single impulse and to ask if he may yield to it without damaging the cultural values which he has created."

Lorenz speaks of the "cultural values which he has created". His use of the word "created" calls attention to the unpredictable contribution of individuals to the development of ethics. This belongs to history and it is hard to see how it can be accounted for in purely biological terms. Whether or not natural selection can produce a being capable of moral reflection, the values which that being recognizes are not themselves a product of natural selection, but of conscious thought. Even if the concept of natural selection can be stretched far enough to account for the moral codes of closed societies, it cannot be made to cover "open morality".

There is, finally, a further complication. "Open morality" in its most striking and influential form was, as we have seen, closely associated with certain religious beliefs. Christians have argued, "God loved you, *therefore* love one another"; and when Christ said "It has been said of old 'love your neighbour, hate your enemy': but I say 'love your enemies'," he added, "you must be perfect, just as your heavenly father is perfect." He did not see himself as creating values but as revealing them. So Christian ethics are based upon a conception of men as children of God, having an eternal destiny. This conception can, of course, be properly regarded from the point of view of the history of ideas as a "cultural value" which man has created. The historian may conveniently leave on one side the question whether the religious beliefs underlying Christian ethics are true or false, for it is not a question which falls within the scope of academic history. But it obviously does not follow that the question cannot be intelligibly raised. One of the great temptations which all academics have to face is that of treating the methodological assumptions of their own discipline as if they were metaphysical truths.

References

Bennett, J. (1967). "Rationality". Humanities Press, New York, U.S.A.

Emmet, D. (1958). "Function, Purpose, and Powers". Macmillan, London, England.

Lorenz, K. (1965). "Man meets Dog". Methuen, London, England.

Lorenz, K. (1967) "On Aggression", Harcourt, Brace and World Inc., New York, U.S.A.

Nadel, S. F. (1953). "Anthropology and Modern Life". Australian National University, quoted by Emmet, op. cit.

Legal Concepts of Responsibility

J. E. HALL WILLIAMS

London School of Economics, London, England

This paper seeks to explain the way in which lawyers approach the problem of legal responsibility, especially in relation to criminal liability. It begins by distinguishing various meanings of responsibility as used in common parlance. This leads to an identification of that meaning of responsibility which is bound up with legal liability and the paper explores the relation between the two. The next subject considered is the conditions which excuse or modify responsibility and the way in which these may be fitted into any general theory, and their rationale. Among lawyers the positive requirements of Intention and Voluntary Action seem to be regarded as necessary preconditions of legal liability. Recent cases on drugs have drawn attention to the grave problems of public policy and individual liberty involved in the interpretation of the offences concerning drugs on a strict basis, excluding the traditional requirements of knowledge or intention.

The moral basis upon which punishment may be justified in such cases is explored. This leads to a general discussion of the different aims of punishment for crime, and the degree to which theories of retribution or reform necessarily involve the notions of moral culpability. The growth of scientific knowledge about the sociological, psychological and social dimensions of human behaviour presents a formidable challenge to traditional views about legal responsibility. The implications for legal theory are considered, and it is suggested that, although the pressures to abandon our legal concepts of responsibility in the face of the growing demands of scientific determinism are very great, as a practical measure if for no other reason (and some of us believe there are other reasons), we must continue to adhere to our beliefs in the concept of the free man, who can deliberate and decide on his conduct and be held accountable for it.

The term "responsibility" exhibits a variety of meanings which must be distinguished in order to identify its proper sense in the criminal law. Professor H. L. A. Hart has delineated four broad categories of responsibility. A sea captain is responsible for the safety of his ship and crew in that by virtue of his position he is under a duty to attend to the welfare of ship and men. This species of responsibility is designated "role responsibility" by Hart. A second type he calls "causal responsibility" which denotes the situation where the expression "is responsible for" may be replaced by the word "caused", thus "the heat was responsible for [or caused] his death". Again, to say of a person that he is "responsible for his actions" is to assert that he has certain normal capacities, namely understanding, reasoning and control of conduct. Hart terms this third variety "capacity responsibility". Fourthly, and most relevant in the present context, is "liability responsibility", either legal or moral.

Whereas it is often assumed that legal responsibility means simply liability to punishment, it is more accurate to say that, although the two concepts overlap, they do not coincide completely. Legal responsibility is concerned with the presence or absence of certain conditions which are mainly psychological in nature. Unless the defendant is legally responsible in this sense, the question of liability does not arise. In contrast, the question of liability includes not merely this enquiry into legal responsibility, but also, for instance, the question whether the conduct was even criminal at all. In sum, legal responsibility is necessary but not sufficient for legal liability. Moral liability-responsibility is similar, such differences as there are originating in the substantive differences between legal rules and moral rules.

Legal responsibility, then, involves an enquiry into whether certain conditions, which are mainly psychological in character, have been satisfied. When one or more of these conditions is not satisfied, the defendant is not regarded as criminally responsible. Applying the deterrent theory of punishment, Bentham described these situations as "cases in which punishment must be inefficacious" and he divided them into two classes. The first class comprised situations in which the defendant was in a continuing state of non-amenability to penal threats, as where he was very young or was insane. The other class covered cases in which the defendant was only beyond deterrence at the specific time of the crime, as where he was acting under a mistake or was drunk. An alternative way of expressing this distinction would be to say that one group of defences caters for the mentally abnormal and the immature, while the other group consists of defences of which the mentally normal and mature can avail themselves.

The two defences available to the mentally abnormal are those of insanity and diminished responsibility. The former defence exculpates the defendant only if his mental disease caused him not to know the true nature of his act or its wrongfulness. It takes no account of persons who have the knowledge required, but still lack the capacity to control their behaviour. This lacuna has now, however, been filled so far as homicide is concerned, by the new plea of diminished responsibility. S. 2 of the Homicide Act 1957 provides that on a murder charge if what is curiously called the "mental responsibility" of the defendant was "substantially impaired" by mental abnormality, he could be convicted not of murder but of manslaughter, carrying a maximum sentence of life imprisonment. The defence is limited in that it only applies to murder and does not excuse from responsibility, but only mitigates the penalty.

The third defence in this class covering persons in a continuing state of non-amenability to penal threats is the defence of infancy, which protects those under ten years of age wholly, and those between ten and fourteen partially, from responsibility.

Of that group of defences available to the mentally normal and mature offender the plea of mistake is perhaps the most common. An honest and reasonable mistake concerning a relevant matter of fact will exculpate the defendant, whereas a mistake of law will not, for everyone is presumed to know the law. There is, secondly, a limited defence of drunkenness which is available in circumstances that favour the situation of the excessive drinker rather than the compulsive alcoholic. The closely related but limited defences of necessity and coercion are designed for those persons who choose to break the law as the lesser of two evils, when faced with an appallingly threatening situation or overwhelming threats from another human agent. The plea of self-defence is available to those who find it necessary to kill in order to preserve themselves or their family from death or serious bodily harm.

The gist of all the defences considered so far is that, although the defendant did the prescribed act, he did it in a state of mind which qualifies him for exculpation. In certain situations, however, the defendant may be able to claim that he did not do the act in any meaningful sense of the phrase. He may have been sleepwalking at the time or have been in a post-epileptic fugue. In such situations the defendant will be able to rely on the defence of automatism and plead that his action was involuntary.

In all these defences the law places the burden of introducing relevant evidence on the defendant, and unless he does so the presumption is that he has the required capacity for responsibility.

What, however, is the rationale of these defences? On what theory of criminal responsibility are they allowed?

One explanation has already been observed in passing. This was Bentham's view that these were cases where punishment was inefficacious because the defendant was not amenable to the threats posed by the criminal law. Professor Hart has dubbed this the theory of "the economy of threats". The argument is, however, vitiated by a non-sequitur. The fact that the defendant could not be deterred by the *threat* of punishment in *his* case does not mean that the actual *administration* of punishment to him would not deter *others*. The punishment of the insane really might help to maintain the efficacy of penal threats for others at its height.

A second view is that moral culpability is a requisite of criminal responsibility which does not exist where the excusing conditions are present. There are two variations of this theory. One approach has found expression in the writings of the American, Professor Jerome Hall, who has written that the essential element in criminal responsibility is "the voluntary doing of a morally wrong act forbidden by penal law". The mistake here is that very many crimes are ethically neutral, particularly minor offences made to further particular social or economic policy. The second approach distinguishes, however, between the moral content of the offence itself and the moral conditions of criminal responsibility. It is not necessary that the offence should be a sin, but it is necessary that the defendant should have deliberately or recklessly broken the law. The defendant can then be said to be morally culpable. However, this requisite of moral blame could no longer be attributed to the defendant if he brought himself within one of the conditions comprised in the defences.

Professor Hart has pushed the analysis a little further, however, and enquired what it is that renders the recognition of these defences an ethical imperative. He believes that the crux of criminal responsibility is the defendant's capacity to conform with the law and his opportunity to exercise that capacity, one or other of which is absent in the situations covered by the defences. This system of criminal responsibility is one within which the defendant can exercise a choice as to whether he obeys the law or not. In the last analysis, however, this rationale of the defences rests on the ethical judgment that society is only justified in punishing those who have had an opportunity of obeying the law which they have rejected.

So far the analysis of legal responsibility has proceeded by way of exclusion; it has been said that if certain conditions are not present, then legal responsibility has been established. Among lawyers, however, the positive analysis of legal responsibility is more fashionable. On this approach legal responsibility consists of what lawyers call *mens rea* or guilty mind, an appropriate form of blameworthiness for every case. The conventional legal analysis is then that this *mens rea* together with the criminal act, *actus reus*, gives rise to criminal liability.

The problems of *mens rea* are more numerous and important than those surrounding the *actus reus* and we must be content to observe of the latter that it is required to be a voluntary act (see automatism above).

It is generally agreed among lawyers that the defendant may be said to have a guilty mind and so be criminally responsible if he did the prescribed act either intentionally or recklessly. Involved in both these states of mind is the notion of foresight of the consequences, in the case of intention the accused not only foresaw but desired the consequences, in the case of recklessness he foresaw the consequences but was careless as to whether they came about or not. It is, however, the element of foresight which lawyers regard as crucial in these two mental states, for the presence of this in the accused is a justification for attributing moral blame to him. Moral culpability is, as already noted, regarded as necessary for criminal responsibility.

Some lawyers hold that negligence is also sufficient for criminal responsibility, and it is the case that some crimes may be committed negligently, but because negligence connotes inadvertence to the consequences of action, other lawyers take the view that the attribution of moral blame is not justified here, with the result that negligence cannot be considered sufficient for criminal responsibility. This analysis, however, omits to mention that also involved in the concept of negligence, besides the notion of inadvertence, is the failure to take such precautions as any reasonable person would have taken in the circumstances. This is surely a justification for blaming the agent concerned.

The error of those who obstruct the entry of negligence into the concept of *mens rea* is the belief that the crux of criminal responsibility is foresight of the consequences. It is suggested, however, that it is rather the capacity to conform to the law and the opportunity to exercise that capacity which is the central concept. It is quite justifiable to attribute blame to those negligent lawbreakers who had both the capacity and the opportunity to exercise the requisite care, as most indeed will have done.

During the nineteenth century, however, there arose in England a species of offence, usually statutory in origin, which did not require *mens rea* at all. All that was required was that the accused should have voluntarily done the prescribed act. It was not necessary that he should have intended or been reckless as to the consequences of his act, nor even that he should have been careless, for the taking of all due care was no defence. This doctrine of strict liability, as it is called, applies today largely to offences created by statute to further particular social or economic policies. It has been the subject of continuous criticism and has recently acquired a wider notoriety in the case of the Oxford schoolteacher, Stephanie Sweet, who was convicted of being concerned in the management of premises which were used for the purpose of smoking cannabis contrary to S. 5 (b) of the Dangerous Drugs Act 1965, despite the prosecution's recognition that the defendant had no knowledge whatsoever that the premises were being so used.*

Before considering the arguments for and against this doctrine we may note that strict liability seems to have prevailed in early societies and to have been significantly related to the status oriented nature of those societies. However, from the very earliest times of recorded English law, and especially between the seventeenth and nineteenth centuries, in England the trend was away from this approach and there is undoubtedly a feeling that the reversal of this trend in the late nineteenth and twentieth centuries represents a severe setback for civilized legal ideals.

It is said that strict liability by its uncompromising attitude to failure to conform to the law ensures a high standard of care and attention to the law's requirements. But it has been doubted how the punishment of a person who was incapable of taking the required precautions is going to be of any value whatsoever. This was the attitude of the Privy Council in the case of *Lim Chin Aik* in 1963. However, this argument is based on a non-sequitur. It is true that the *threat* of punishment is clearly ineffective in cases where persons are not capable of conforming to the law at the time of the offence, but it does not follow from this that the actual *application* of punishment to the defendant may not cause *other* persons—and indeed the defendant himself—to be more careful in their behaviour in future.

Surely the real objection to the doctrine is not a utilitarian but an ethical one. For under this doctrine defendants are punished irrespective of their capacity to conform to the law and opportunity to exercise that capacity. Thus, the doctrine violates the fundamental requirements of criminal responsibility at common law, which, as has been seen, rests ultimately on an ethical base.

Somewhat akin to strict liability and equally objectionable is the doctrine of vicarious liability. Normally in criminal law the minimum condition for liability is that the defendant should have committed the prescribed act himself. But in exceptional cases one person may be held responsible for the criminal behaviour of another. Thus a master may in certain situations be liable for the crimes of his servants, even though they were committed without his knowledge and against his orders.

This review of responsibility in the criminal law would not be com-

* On appeal to the House of Lords, after the Divisional Court had confirmed the conviction of Miss Sweet, it was held that the offence in question did not involve strict liability but required proof of *mens rea*; the prosecution must prove the knowledge of the defendant. (1969). Crim. L.R. 189, *The Times*, January 24, 1969.

plete without an examination of the relation between notions of responsibility and the aims of punishment. The English penal system is not dominated by any particular penal aim, but rather by an amalgam of aims, consisting of retribution, deterrence, and reform. Retribution is a backward looking approach in that the punishment is justified solely by reference to the evil act of the defendant involved in the commission of the crime. Deterrence and reform look to the future. The utilitarian theory of deterrence holds that punishment, which is in itself an evil, can be justified if it deters the individual defendant from offending again or deters other potential offenders. The reformatory approach is geared solely to curing the offender of his anti-social tendencies. What bearing do these theories have on notions of responsibility?

One illustration must suffice. The retributive approach clearly postulates that the offender has voluntarily done something morally wrong. But how dependent on the penal aim of retribution is this principle that moral culpability is a prerequisite to punishment? Some modern thinkers believe that its retention is no longer justifiable after the demise of retributive ideas. Thus Baroness Wootton of Abinger has urged that we should abandon all current notions of responsibility and attempts to assign blame and concentrate instead on the reform of persons manifesting anti-social behaviour. The only prerequisite for subjecting people to this kind of reformative treatment should be that they have committed a proscribed act irrespective, however, of the state of mind in which it was done. The kind of investigation that is pursued at present in order to establish *mens rea* should be left till the post-conviction stage and merely considered as one of the factors determining the appropriate treatment.

Nevertheless, it is suggested that conviction of a crime in accordance with present notions of responsibility can be supported as a prerequisite to punishment on ethical grounds quite independent of retributive ideas. As has been seen, the most convincing rationale of current notions of criminal responsibility is that a person should not be punished unless he had the capacity to obey the law and the opportunity to exercise that capacity and yet nevertheless chose to commit the crime. This can still be urged as an *ethically imperative* requirement even under a system devoted to the reform of the offender. It is so regarded because of our respect for human rights and the freedom of individuals. Our interference with such freedom should be limited to those occasions when someone has freely put himself at risk of being dealt with for his deeds.

This kind of attack on criminal responsibility is not so easily repulsed, however, for the rising tide of determinist ideas has increasingly called in question the existing conceptions of responsibility, plainly based as they are on an assumption of free will. The burden of this attack is that the present distinctions drawn between those who have the capacity to obey the law and those who do not are totally artificial, because it is probable that those who are supposedly capable of controlling their conduct by choice are in fact just as incapable of such choice as are those who are recognized not to have this capacity. Their decisions and choices are determined by the events which preceded them.

The usual reaction of lawyers is to evade rather than grapple with this issue. The evidence and extent of support for deterministic ideas are belittled and shelter is sought behind the presumption in favour of free will. The answer to the onslaught of determinism is not as far to seek as the behaviour of such lawyers would suggest, however. The crux of the present conception of criminal responsibility is the capacity to obey the law and the opportunity to exercise that capacity. If a person deliberates about committing an offence and decides not to, he can quite justifiably describe what he has made as a choice; he will obtain satisfaction from making it, and he will be able to predict in consequence that there will be no interference with his person by the law. Surely, under any conceivable system of determinism these choices remain choices and these satisfactions remain satisfactions, even if the choices are determined and even if other factors besides the choices condition the satisfaction.

In discussions of determinism and legal responsibility it is usually psychological and sociological determinism which is in question. But there are scholars who have urged the importance of biological factors in the explanation of crime. This approach to the aetiology of criminal behaviour began with Cesare Lombroso, the Italian scholar, who in his book "L'Uomo Delinquente" first published in 1876 expounded his theory of the born criminal. Lombroso urged the existence of a distinct anthropological type, who was likely or even bound to commit crime and who was characterized by certain malformations of the skull and skeleton as well as by other physical stigmata of degeneration.

Lombroso's theory was subjected to severe criticism by Dr. Charles Goring, an English prison doctor, in his book "The English Convict" published in 1919, and an attempted vindication of the theory by the American Ernest Hooton in 1939 failed to make much impression.

A more sophisticated development occurred with the attempt to establish a link between bodily endowment and personality and to relate this typology with criminal behaviour. The pioneer here was the German psychiatrist Ernst Kretschmer who was followed in the U.S.A. by William H. Sheldon. In his "Varieties of Delinquent Youth" Sheldon described how he found a preponderance of the athletic physique among his delinquent sample, a type characterized by adventure and aggression.

The latest and most refined study in this line is that by the Gluecks described in "Physique and Delinquency" (1956). These authors correlated physical type with various psychological and sociocultural factors in an attempt to arrive at syndromes of criminogenic factors.

Despite the contemptuous dismissals of this approach by sociologists such as Edwin H. Sutherland, one may feel that there is truth in Sheldon's fundamental proposition that "behaviour is a function of structure". But it must be recognized that the implications of this work are deterministic in that it postulates the existence of a psycho-physical type endowed by heredity with a disposition to criminality.

A not dissimilar result has been arrived at in England by a psychologist of the Behaviourist School, H. J. Eysenck. He claims likewise to have identified a hereditarily determined constellation of traits associated with criminality. The criminal is characterized by the mesomorphic or athletic physique as suggested by Sheldon and the Gluecks and exhibits poor psychomotor control. Neurotic tendencies and extraversion are the third and fourth significant factors, the extravert being less amenable to conditioning which is the fifth trait in the constellation. This theory again heavily emphasizes the hereditary approach to criminality.

Finally, considerable interest has been aroused by evidence emerging of the significance of chromosome imbalance in the aetiology of crime. In the 1967 Annual Report of the Medical Research Council it is reported, on the basis of evidence gathered in a study of psychopaths at the State Hospital, Carstairs, that a male with an extra male chromosome is over six feet tall, seldom normal enough to account for his actions and possibly predisposed to criminal behaviour. This type would only account for a small proportion of criminals, specifically those committing "a succession of apparently motiveless crimes, mostly against property". American and Norwegian studies seem to confirm this.

There is a more impressive body of evidence for the significance of the biological factor in crime than many sociologically oriented scholars are prepared to acknowledge. But it certainly does not justify any theory of biological determinism on Lombrosian lines, which would undermine the basis of current conceptions of criminal responsibility. Moreover, the law must continue to base its notions of legal liability on the assumption of a person having had a free choice as regards his behaviour. This is one of the notions which we must adhere to as a matter of expediency even if we no longer have such firm conviction about it as our ancestors. But this does not prevent the laws from moving in the direction which modern science points when it comes to dealing with extreme cases of personality disorder and those whose conduct is clearly pathological or immature. In sentencing at least, these factors are becoming increasingly recognized as of material significance.

One of the justifications today of deterrent sentences is that they influence public opinion and help to reinforce moral standards. The evidence for this is slight, and there are some indications that standards and moral judgments are not influenced by the law in the short run. But the amenability of persons to punishment is clearly affected by their personality and we are presently exploring the psychological dimensions of the personality which may be significant in this connection.

Sociologists meanwhile are currently developing theories about self concept and role definition which may in turn provide new clues for those concerned with the administration of criminal justice.

ACKNOWLEDGEMENT

The author wishes to acknowledge the great help received in the preparation of this paper from his research assistant, Mr. J. P. W. Cartwright, LL.B.

REFERENCES

Eysenck, H. J. (1964). "Crime and Personality". Houghton Mifflin, Boston, U.S.A.

Glueck, Sheldon Eleanor. (1956). "Physique and Delinquency". Harper, New York.

Goring, C. (1919). "The English Convict". H.M.S.O. (abridged edition.)

Hall, J. (1960). "General Principles of Criminal Law". 2nd Ed. Bobbs-Merrill, Indianapolis.

Hart, H. L. A. (1968). "Punishment and Responsibility". Clarendon Press, Oxford.

Hooton, E. A. (1939). "Crime and the Man". Harvard University Press, Cambridge, Mass.

Kretschmer, E. (1936). "Physique and Character". Kegan Paul, London. Harcourt Brace and World, New York.

Lombroso, C. (1876). "L'Uomo Delinquente".

Sheldon, W. H. (1949). "Varieties of Delinquent Youth". Harper, New York.

Sutherland, E. H. (1955). "Principles of Criminology" (5th ed. revised by Donald R. Cressey). University of Chicago Press.

Wootton, B. (1963). "Crime and Criminal Law" Stevens, London.

Guilt and Responsibility—Feelings or Reality?

D. A. POND

Department of Psychiatry, London Hospital Medical College, London, England

INTRODUCTION

This paper will largely deal with individual guilt and responsibility rather than with collective guilt and responsibility. Following a suggestion first made by Father Victor White, the eminent Roman Catholic priest and student of Jungian psychology, one may usefully contrast the two main senses in which the word guilt is used.

GUILT AS AN OBJECTIVE STATE

For example, for the lawyer, guilt implies an offence against the law; for the moralist an offence against certain principles; for the theologian a sin, an offence against God. However, for all these three, as well as for most people who use the word guilty, there is implied not only the commission of a certain act, but also a certain state of mind in the person doing the act, which indicates the conscious intention to commit the offence. This state of mind is connected with the second use of the word.

SUBJECTIVE EMOTIONAL STATE

Psychologists and psychiatrists use the word not so much for the above objective situations, the commissions of certain acts, but to describe a subjective emotional state—a sense of wrongdoing—that need not necessarily arise when the law or morals are transgressed or a sin committed. On the one hand, no sense of guilt may be present in a man, before, during or after the commission of a serious crime; and in contrast there are many people who lead blameless lives and yet are covered with a profound guilt sense into which they may have more or less fluctuating insight. Sometimes this morbid sense of guilt is easily recognized for what it is, as in the severely depressed patient convinced that he has committed the unforgiveable sin, is responsible for all the world's ills, or is under some other obvious delusion. Yet even in these serious cases tragedies sometimes unavoidably occur, such as when a patient butchers his own family, convinced that thereby he is saving

55

them from the tortures of hell that he has caused them to suffer. In other patients, the sense of guilt may be more subtly disturbed, and can sometimes paradoxically result in persistent grossly anti-social and even delinquent behaviour.

The ontogenetic beginnings of the sense of guilt have been traced back earlier and earlier in the development of the human personality. In particular, Melanie Klein claims that it originates from the early months of life when the baby is already aware of intense and primitive aggression towards itself and the environment (especially mother) which it tries to control unavailingly. A paralyzing and irrational sense of guilt can be found early on in children, and in some it may persist more or less unchanged into adult life (resulting in crippling symptoms if not anti-social or other abnormal behaviour that concerns others). An important problem to be solved in the upbringing of children is how to maintain a proper and flexible sense of guilt so that it is not disastrously bound up to minutae of children's behaviour. Even nowadays a morbid sense of guilt may become attached to masturbation accompanying other sexual disturbances, but the effect of making pre-genital sources of satisfaction guilt laden is even more serious and can result in adults having no real capacity to behave according to adult standards. On the other hand, of course, adult values of right and wrong behaviour and thought change, and we have to allow for an individual's conscience in the sense of that part of him which can rationally adjust to his or her own sense of right and wrong.

There are many difficulties if responsibility is analysed in a way similar to that of guilt; that is, by considering it first in relationship to an objective state on the one hand, and secondly to a subjective experience on the other. The word has a much wider connotation than guilt; it is concerned not only with actions of all sorts (not just those proscribed by lawyer, moralist or theologian) but also with anticipated actions, plans and thoughts. These are matters outside the legal province, and, many would argue, largely outside the scope of scientific investigation as well.

In contrast to the legal use of guilt, in that a man is innocent until proved guilty, the law and most people in everyday relationships assume that a man is responsible until proved otherwise. Age (both young and old) and infirmity of mind (for example, in terms of mental capacity) are limiting factors that are sometimes taken into account. But it will be noted that the ultimate limits of these factors are set arbitrarily by society's own standards which have varied notably throughout the ages. For example, the age at which criminal proceedings can be taken against children has been progressively raised, and the age of responsibility as regards consent to marry, etc. progressively lowered. Chronological age is in fact only broadly related to responsibility.

The subjective sense of responsibility is hedged round with even more psychological pitfalls than the sense of guilt. Everyone knows the sense in which one says, "It's none of my business" as a means of denying responsibility for someone else's behaviour about which we have mixed feelings. On the other hand, there is very commonly in some people an excessive sense of responsibility; for example, the boss who can't delegate functions, the overprotective mother, and the general tendency of some people to organize things in order to cut down their own anxiety. The mature adult is not necessarily one who has a maximal subjective sense of responsibility, nor one who actively involves himself in every claim upon his "duty".

The following factors are the main ones that appear to set some limits to personal responsibility for one's own actions and thoughts:

COLLECTIVE OR SOCIAL FACTORS

(a) *Actual incapability.* For example, man is not responsible for the weather.

(b) *Ignorance.* This may at times be the result of deliberate concealment by others; for example, citizens' actions in war-time, though one has to recognize that there is a positive duty upon people to find out the truth as far as possible.

INTRAPERSONAL FACTORS

(a) *Lack of intelligence and knowledge.* For example, the subnormal adult.

(b) *Inadequate or wrong motivation.* This concept leads to the problem of the unconscious determination of activity, evidence of which is easier to accept in minor matters than major ones; for example, the everyday slips of the tongue so brilliantly described in Freud's Psychopathology of Everyday Life. What is meant by the Will, guilty intention and other such terms in legal and everyday use have surprisingly and sadly not been matters of much interest to psychologists and psychiatrists. One suspects that both groups implicitly if not explicitly confuse Will with Free-will, and an implied antithesis to that scientific determinism which is the indispensable basis of laboratory and clinical investigation. Hence perhaps many of us hope the problem will disappear if the sciences of human behaviour progress far enough—a not very realistic or sensible attitude on the whole.

(c) *Other character traits or personality characteristics.* These are of

significance in exemplifying the ways in which anxiety is dealt
with; for example, by dissociation, as in hysteria, or by obsessive-
compulsive mechanisms.

COLLECTIVE   GUILT   AND   RESPONSIBILITY—SPECIAL   INTERACTIONS
BETWEEN SOCIAL AND INTRAPERSONAL FACTORS

One of the main difficulties in talking about personal responsibility as
if it were a unitary trait is that not only do people vary between themselves in their subjective sense of responsibility and the actual amount
of responsible behaviour they show, but the same person differs from
time to time and from place to place, both in the subjective and
objective senses of the word responsible. Some degree of "irrational"
social cohesion is necessary for society to hang together at all. It may be
harmless enough, for example, when it involves fashions in clothes, but
the so-called power of suggestion can be invoked to describe, if not
explain, all sorts of behaviour. Life would indeed be intolerable and
impossible if one had to think out everything from scratch. Collective
guilt or corporate responsibility are terms often used to describe the
thoughts and actions of groups, or more often to make claims of what
they ought to do and think. Much was heard of collective guilt during
the Nazi war crimes trials, and social groups are often urged to assume
more responsibility for the actions of their own members (for example,
when a medical staff committee has to deal with an indiscretion—a
breach of professional conduct by one of its members). People, whether
singly or in groups, are also urged to feel responsible for the sufferings of
others less fortunate than themselves (for example, refugees or victims
of poverty or prejudice) when there may be no legal or other contractual
obligation. A child comes across such demands when the whole class is
kept in as a punishment for the misdemeanours of one or more of its
members (and not only when this is the simplest rough-and-ready
justice for a teacher who can't find out the true culprits). The family
(whatever its actual size and composition) is of course the earliest and
most important small group in which the formation and isolation of
tensions moulds the character of the children and allows their differentiation into separate adults to a greater or lesser extent.

The ambiguities underlying many of these situations have often been
brought out in literature and drama as well as by moral philosophers.
The psychiatrist's special view of collective guilt and responsibility
rests only on his knowledge and experience of behaviour of patients in
families, group psychotherapy and hospital communities. In these
situations, the interaction between the internal psychological conflicts
of the patients and their overt common attitudes and behaviour can be

minutely analysed and more easily altered. One can see persons acting out roles, such as the group scapegoat, without their necessarily being consciously aware of doing so, or why such roles satisfy their own internal needs. The lack of a 1 : 1 relationship between the subjective sense of responsibility for action, and the objective role cast on them may be startling. Intelligence, as conventionally understood or measured by tests, has little to do with self-awareness in such situations. One of the most extreme and dangerous situations in which almost all people may act irresponsibly, in ways unlike their usual behaviour and with subsequent guilt and shame, is in a rioting crowd. The mob is a primitive psychological horde that few can resist once actually in it.

The individual differences between the degrees of responsibility shown by people and by the same person from time to time and from place to place, are also shown in animals, though to a minor degree. Every breeder recognizes the virtually untrainable dog in a pack, and the elderly rogue elephant is rejected by the rest of the herd on the sound biological principle of preserving the rest of them. Most of this variation between members of the same species is environmental in origin, some genetic and some the result of injury, usually to the higher parts of the central nervous system. However, one must not forget that the non-conforming individual is of positive evolutionary value, and the role of the biological sport in adapting to changing environments is, of course, recognized by every biologist. Responsibility is not therefore shown by only socially conforming behaviour, and there is an important sense in which nobody can finally judge the rightness of many pieces of behaviour, which is why all mature societies recognize the conscientious objector.

SOME IMPLICATIONS

The individual differences between people as regards the responsibility that they can take and have taken is a matter that must be much more allowed for in penology and education at present. Baroness Wootton is doubtless right in her strictures against the very notion of responsibility as currently employed in legal procedures. A sense of responsibility is not proportional to the seriousness of the crime, either in the popular estimate of the seriousness of what is committed, or in the scale of punishment in the penal code. Society takes far too lightly dangerously irresponsible driving "under the influence", and no-one can say that a prisoner feels that a sentence of ten years means a crime twice as serious as that for which he might get five years, or that twice the length of the sentence passed means the need for twice as much reform. The assessment of how best to re-train a man relies little on his subjective sense of responsibility but more on other character traits, such as intelligence, tolerance anxiety, rapidity of learning new habits, presence of adequate motivation to change, etc. It must be admitted that psychologists and psychiatrists have no satisfactory working classification of personality appropriate for the even relatively limited aims of penology. More research is needed into the genetic and environmental factors which interact with each other to produce that right degree of responsibility in adult affairs that is implied by the term, the mature adult.

It is a paradox that Freud made the great advances in psychotherapy as a result of understanding unconscious mechanisms by his assumption that apparently irrational processes, like dreams, are determined in the same sense as we speak of physical phenomena being determined. The paradox is that the assumption of determinism results in a greater degree of the sense of free will, and also of a greater sense of personal responsibility. Increasing the area of responsibility for one's own actions implies overcoming some sort of internal block, and the process is similar to that by which a child learns to walk: the first steps have to be taken before the action can actually be done properly. Tasks have to be graded and there is an important sense in which responsibility is conferred on people rather than earned or innately acquired. There is no clear correlation between the objective ability to be responsible and the subjective sense of being responsible, though this sense can undoubtedly act as a motivating influence in certain social situations. Lastly, one may distinguish between the sociological and the psychological problems of the nature of authority. Much is being written at the moment about the decline of traditional authorities and yet the need for some overall sense of an absolute (for a recent expression of this consider Conor Cruse O'Brien's book on the religious role of the United Nations). From the psychological and psychiatric point of view, one is mainly interested in the way that the nature and power of this overriding authority is communicated to the child through the mediation of the family.

Discussion

BROUGHTON: I should like to take up Professor Mitchell's point about the lack of selective advantage of "open" morality—or "closed" too, for that matter—to a society or species. Whilst either of these might itself be selectively neutral, surely it could also be an obligatory consequence of the evolution of thought processes which could themselves have had selective advantages at lower levels—to the individual.

MITCHELL: It is reasonable to assume that such characteristics as intelligence and sympathy are (a) of selective advantage to the individual, and (b) a necessary condition of advance from the "closed" to the "open" morality. It is not clear, however, that they are also a sufficient condition of that advance as the expression "obligatory consequence" suggests. No doubt people who are intelligent and sympathetic have it in them to develop an open morality, but large numbers have not done so, because there was nothing in their cultural tradition to encourage it. There may be a sense in which there is "natural selection" between cultural traditions, but it must be distinguished from genetic selection.

POOLE: It seems paradoxical that, whilst behaviour which resembles human ethical behaviour occurs in animals, we are not prepared to talk of a courageous ant or baboon; this would generally be regarded as anthropomorphism. The fact that a similar kind of behaviour occurs in both men and animals suggests an underlying similarity of mechanism. Surely the difference between animal and human courage is that a man who rescues another human being from drowning can foresee the consequences of his act of courage in terms of the risk he is taking whilst, as far as we know, an animal cannot do this. The difference therefore is that a human being can refuse to act courageously whilst an animal cannot. The active choice to act in this way is what gives a human act of self sacrifice its merit.

MITCHELL: I agree that this is the most important difference. A further one is that the ability of human beings to conceptualize means that they can be acting courageously when their actual overt behaviour is of a kind which, if it occurred in an animal, would not be regarded as "courageous" at all, e.g. turning the other cheek.

DE REUCK: Bravery may well be a virtue inherited biologically, but knowledge of the occasions on which it is proper to be brave is part of our cultural inheritance. For example, twentieth century Christians would no longer think it right to embark on a crusade.

WOODRUFF: Professor Pond has referred to scientific determinism as the underlying assumption in all laboratory and clinical investigation. I suspect that the majority of people here today would agree. Yet we are assembled to discuss ethical responsibility and this concept in my view is logically incompatible with scientific determinism. I wonder whether Professor Pond can resolve the paradox.

POND: Professor Woodruff's question requires more philosophical knowledge than I possess to answer properly. Determinism *v.* Indeterminism is one part of an argument going on in the physical sciences for at least 40 years, and it is important to stress that we are making an *assumption*, not accepting an axiom or fact, when talking about strict determinism. Everyday experience of ourselves gives evidence that without the equally unproven *assumption* of personal responsibility for at least most of one's actions and thoughts, society would rapidly grind to a halt and in that pragmatic sense, if no other, some sort of free-will is as proven (or unproven) as determinism. The interesting fact is that by assuming that apparently irrational behaviour can be investigated and "understood" if not "explained", Freud started a whole series of methods of treatment which led to people having more personal responsibility, judged both by their behaviour as seen by others, and by their subjective experience of decision-making.

PRINGLE: Could a sense of guilt be necessary for the development of social behaviour? Might the tendency to feel guilt be genetically controlled?

HUMPHREY: To what extent does Dr. Pond regard such emotions as disgust, horror and pity as socially conditioned? My reason for asking is that it seems to me possible that they may once have played an important role—and to some extent may still do so today—in limiting fighting between individuals, and in acting as a socially cohesive force. The person whose "stomach turns" at the sight of another wounded human being or who faints at the sight of blood is not so uncommon, and a sense of pity for the individual in the sights of a rifle may, for example, cause a soldier purposely to aim badly. Although such emotions are obviously socially conditioned in part, do they also correspond to some extent to the factors which limit conflict between animals of the same species, and if so might they not have been subject to positive selection during the evolution of the human race? If so, it seems likely that a serious weakening of the force of such emotions in limiting conflicts will occur once the person who uses a weapon does not see with his own eyes the immediate consequences of his action. The man who fires a long-range howitzer, or who presses the button of a nuclear missile, will require imagination to picture what the consequences will be at the receiving end. I suppose, indeed, that one of the aims of military training is to depict the enemy as a depersonalized object of hate or fear rather than as a fellow human being, and to expel such feelings of pity so far as he is concerned. I have never understood how the Christian churches managed to reconcile themselves to this.

POND: I will answer Professor Pringle's and Dr. Humphrey's points together. The genetic contribution to the structure of personality is undeniable, though its importance relative to learning and environmental experience has been played down in recent years. However, we cannot identify any particular aspect of personality which is even predominantly genetically controlled. The particular objects, or pieces of behaviour, which arouse emotion are learned by the influence of the environment. There is almost certainly in the human no such thing as, for example, an "innate" fear of snakes or guilt about incest. Thus, what arouses our disgust, horror or pity is socially conditioned, or rather mainly family conditioned. Unfortunately, the adult and socially significant things which should arouse such emotions if we are to enlist public sympathy for their eradication, can only be properly comprehended by older children or adults, years after the strength of such emotions have been fully developed and often already fixed to highly personal, usually bodily, and socially comparatively less important pieces of behaviour, such as the mechanisms of excretion and auto-erotic activity. The imbalance between the strength of the emotions and the forces developing in the child to control them or to defend itself against them, leads to battles that are perceived, by the pre-school child particularly, as fearful struggles. The bad inside oneself is dealt with by denial, projection, repression and other mechanisms which can all too easily become the means whereby the bad outside oneself, especially that in others, is managed.

Ethologists have given a new twist to the debate about the social value of man's emotional life, but it is of interest to note that, for example, Lorenz and W. M. S. Russell come to fairly opposite conclusions about the place of aggression in the human species. Though there is some evidence of assortative non-random mating within some groups (e.g. Professors' wives tend to be more intelligent than dustmen's spouses) which can lead to markedly skew distribution of intelligence in the resulting children, I doubt if the human race's total mixture of genes (even those affecting intelligence) has been much changed by selection since civilization began. We have still to deal with the same old Adam with primitive drives and limited imagination, which characteristics are more randomly distributed in the population than intelligence.

PRINGLE: Could all feelings of guilt be absent from an individual?

POND: One sees abnormal characters who appear to have no subjective sense of guilt, as judged by their own utterances, and no capacity to learn from being conventionally punished; nor any evidence that they would even obey the code of "honour among thieves". There is strong evidence that such people have grown up in impersonal institutions or emotionally deprived families; there is nothing to suggest that they have a "constitutional" absence of the capacity to develop a sense of guilt.

DE BEUCK: What evidence there is might suggest that the effect of existing moral codes could well be to the detriment of the human genetic pool. Even if it is uncertain whether or not welfare economics is in fact doing genetic damage to our race by encouraging the less intelligent sections of the community to have disproportionately too many children, it is clear that modern medical skills allied to welfare ethics keep alive many people of genetically inferior stock who not long ago would have died before they reached reproductive age. Most attempts to modify the moral code in order to put it on a "sound evolutionary basis', by for example introducing eugenic concepts which in effect grade people according to the "value" of their genes, seem like a leap from the frying pan into the fire. Perhaps we do not need to choose between a compassionate ethic valuing the highest possible development of every individual (and incidentally favouring the widest genetic diversity) and a more efficient ethic placing a higher value on genes than on individual people and stressing the future at the expense of the present. Perhaps the answer is to suggest that the greater part of the burden of the human evolutionary process has already—for the past half million years—been transferred from the biological to the cultural mode; and to look forward to the day when the two modes will be re-united by man's culturally acquired ability to repair damaged genes.

POND: It is important to care for all men, however physically damaged or psychologically depraved they may be, but I believe it is no part of caring for them as human beings to say they have the right to breed freely. However, I believe the current danger is not so much that the less intelligent sections of the community have disproportionately too many children, since there is increasing evidence that universal knowledge of simple contraceptive measures, coupled with the chances of economic improvement, lead to small families in almost all social classes and levels of intelligence. The more serious danger is well described in Michael Young's, "The New Meritocracy", amongst other places; that is, social stratification based on "real" differences of ability and personality and not in privileges of birth, education, family pressure, etc. At the present time we see the poor are poorer and the rich richer, intellectually, and the social consequences of this have yet to be worked out (though adumbrated in Aldous Huxley's "Brave New World").

MASON: I have been dazzled by the displays of donnishness and expertise in the papers, but I still have not heard what ethics are or what they are for. Are they, as I suspect, a set of tricks imposed on the young by the old in the name of a quiet life and isn't contemporary parental dismay largely because the young, having got economic power for the first time in history, are in a position to reject our particular "set of tricks"? There are, and have been, so many ethical systems that we need a yard stick to evaluate them. Would you accept Waddington's yardstick of wisdom or common sense and, if so, what is common and what is sensible for now?

POND: Criticizing adolescents for the same reasons as we do today is well documented at least as far back as Socrates and the Old Testament, and the young have always seen through the pretensions of their parents' generation. "By their fruits" is the only possible pragmatic evaluation of different systems of ethics, but we can still discuss what sorts of fruits we want. There is perhaps now more of a dialogue between the generations on these topics than there was in most previous ages, and I think that this is a good thing.

Bisexuality and Ethics

RICHARD P. MICHAEL

Department of Psychiatry, Institute of Psychiatry,
University of London, London, England

INTRODUCTION

Our sexual proclivities can cause trouble. Strong views are held by many of us on what constitutes an acceptable pattern of sexual behaviour, and we may (or may not) abjure in our private lives what we proscribe for others. Support for a particular view-point is sought from whatever source is to hand—from philosophy, ethics, religion, the law and other social institutions and, more recently, even from biology—where useful data is at last beginning to replace mere speculation and hypothesis.

My task is to put before you some of the biological data that are currently emerging about bisexuality and to consider their possible bearing on the human situation. This is a restricted objective. I do not propose to deal with the clinical problem of homosexuality because no brief, superficial treatment of this subject is ever useful.

For present purposes, by bisexuality I mean the manifestation or expression of sexual behaviour that is usually characteristic of the opposite sex; the emphasis here being upon the behavioural aspects. There is no doubt that the prospect of an otherwise apparently healthy woman strapping an artificial phallus to herself and performing the male role with another woman, or, equally, that of a man dressing in female undergarments and simulating the female role, causes an intense emotional reaction in the public mind.

Although comparative anthropology informs us that activities of this kind have been found in widely diverse human cultures from antiquity, the reactions they evoke in some of us are so strongly aversive that the phenomenology of that which is to be evaluated becomes distorted. This rather widespread inability to deal with the phenomenon is expressed by the failure even to index the topic in many otherwise authoritative works on ethics; and the confusion of terminology and of value judgements to be found in the writings of so prominent a theologian as Karl Barth may be similarly accounted for. But it is not a part of my present aim to consider either the sources of this discomfort and distaste or the dimly conscious motivations of those, including myself, who feel the need to express opinions on these topics.

BISEXUAL BEHAVIOUR IN INFRA-HUMAN MAMMALS

The experimental investigation of freaks like the free-martin, a condition occurring in dizygotic twin calves with some degree of anastomosis between their placental circulations, during the First World War, initiated an era of intense activity in this field of experimental biology. Intersex conditions have since been produced genetically, by grafting gonads and by hormone treatments, and are familiar to all biologists.

What is, apparently, much less well known is the extent to which bisexual patterns of behaviour are represented in the *normal* behavioural repertoire of many untreated mammals. Thus, normally oestrous rats and guinea-pigs will frequently show mounting activity, directed towards other females and males, when in maximum heat. This behaviour is used and scored by experimental psychologists when making quantitative measures of the intensity of oestrous behaviour. When two female cats are at the height of oestrus one may mount the other in a manner characteristic of the male and execute a series of male-like pelvic thrusts, yet both females will be fully receptive if immediately paired with an active tom cat. In other circumstances, normal males will mount other normal male cats and the initiative can be altered by altering the territorial situation and the conditions under which the tests are conducted. Many similar examples could be cited by those concerned with animal husbandry, particularly in cattle, pigs and horses.

I am not attempting here to make any direct analogy with the human situation, but bisexual behavioural patterns are also seen with considerable frequency among the infra-human primates. In a recent, well-intentioned and otherwise well-informed book on Christian ethics and sex (Roy, 1968), one reads that "animals, especially the primates, do not engage in homosexual relations except when they become domesticated", and that "certain of the primates, however, frequently have homosexual encounters when confined in a zoo or circus". Such beliefs as these are widely held even among the educated although they are not in accord with the biological facts. Altmann (1962 and personal communication) has records of some 200 homosexual encounters in baboons and macaques observed in the wild. But the view persists that these behaviour patterns are somehow "unnatural", occurring only as distortions in adverse environmental situations imposed by man. The male rhesus monkey shows a cycle of mounting towards the female with a peak in activity at about the time of the female's ovulation. Some 20% of all females studied by us under laboratory conditions also show a cycle of mounting activity, *directed towards the male*, also with maxima at about the time of ovulation (Michael, 1968). Some males tolerate being mounted in this way by females, others do not.

There are numerous references in both field and laboratory studies to these bisexual patterns of behaviour being observed in both the male and female of many primate species. In the well known review by Ford and Beach (1951), in only 28 of the 76 human societies studied were homosexual activities absent, rare or carried on in secrecy, and sociological data indicate that some 30% of adult American and British males have had some homosexual experience.

If it is conceded that Man, as a species, carries the weight of an evolutionary past on his shoulders, such data are to be predicted. Nevertheless, so far as I am aware, it is only for *us* that "earthquakes, famine, pestilence, saracens, floods and very fat, voracious field mice" are confidently anticipated as unwelcome sequelae—to quote from Benedict Carpzov's "Practica Rerum Criminalium". Although, more sadly, imprisonment for up to sixty years is still the penalty in one American State for homosexual activity between consenting adults in private.

RECENT EXPERIMENTAL FINDINGS

It has been known for some years that the administration of gonadal sex hormones during certain phases of embryonic and early post-natal development alters the appearance of both the external genitalia and internal accessory sex structures while, generally, in mammals, the gonads themselves remain little affected. Thus, the exposure of genetically female guinea-pigs during foetal life to androgen—by administering testosterone propionate to the pregnant mothers—results in varying degrees of external masculinization and pseudo-hermaphroditism.

It has been discovered more recently that exposing the embryonic female to androgen in this way impairs its capacity subsequently to exhibit the normal pattern of female behaviour and augments aspects of behaviour normally characteristic of genetic males. These changes in the behavioural repertoire only become manifest after puberty when sexual maturity is reached. Without describing these well-known studies in too great detail, what is important here is, firstly, that permanent, irreversible effects upon behaviour are produced which only become expressed after a long intervening period of development, and secondly, that the androgen must be administered during a certain *critical* period in embryonic development, for after this sensitive period has passed no permanent changes can be produced.

It happens in mammals that the basic, anhormonal somatotype is female, the homogametic sex, and the evidence at present available indicates that it is the presence of androgens that cause maleness, while their absence, rather than the presence of oestrogens, results in femaleness. It follows that the administration of oestrogen to genetic males during embryogenesis does not have an equal and opposite effect to that of androgen on genetic females. This should be mentioned because I have already been guilty of over-simplification.

These studies have developed in two interesting directions. Firstly, attention has now been given to sex-related behavioural patterns, that is those not primarily concerned with copulation. Brief periods of hormone treatments during early development produce permanent changes in such sexually dimorphic behaviour as cyclic running activity in rats, activity in open-field tests, the pattern of micturition of dogs, as well as changes in general body growth, in pituitary function, and in oxygen consumption, where this is sexually dimorphic (as in the guinea-pig). These changes in the organism are altogether too pervasive to be accounted for simply by the associated external masculinization occurring in these experimentally produced pseudohermaphrodites and the enlargement of the clitoris into a phallus.

The second interesting and important development has depended upon the extension of these studies to primates—with their long gestation period, complex social organizations and immensely enhanced neocortical development. Goy (1968) and his colleagues at the Oregon Regional Primate Centre have now successfully produced pseudo-hermaphroditism in a small group of genetically female rhesus monkeys by treating the mothers with androgen during pregnancy. Experiments such as these require considerable patience since one must wait five or more years for the infants to attain maturity, but interesting changes in the behaviour of this masculinized group have already been recorded during the first few years of their development. What, it may be asked, have these studies to do with human bisexuality? Well, all these genetic females show more *threat behaviour*, more *rough and tumble play*, more *play initiation*, more *chasing* and more *mounting activity*, than a group of control females studied concurrently. These results strongly indicate that the whole "personality" of these developing primates has been influenced in a male direction by the change in their hormonal environment at a critical period during their intra-uterine development.

Can such chemical influences as these be operative during human embryonic development? Money (1968) and his associates at Johns Hopkins have recently given fresh attention to these problems by studying three clinical syndromes in which the pre-natal hormonal environment of the human foetus has been upset, namely: progestin-induced pseudohermaphroditism, female hyperadrenocortical pseudo-hermaphroditism (the congenital adrenogenital syndrome), and Turner's syndrome. The first of these—the progestin-induced condition—occurs as the result of the administration of progestational agents with androgenic activity early in pregnancy in an effort to prevent a miscarriage. The second is associated with a recessive genetic trait requiring life-long control with cortisone. In both conditions the human foetus is exposed to excess androgen and external masculinization results. In Turner's syndrome, which is due to a genetic defect, typically an absent sex chromosome, the gonads, on the other hand, are missing entirely: in the absence of any foetal gonadal hormones, the basic psychosexual differentiation is female. Money and his colleagues have compared these conditions using the following seven categories of psychosexual difference: the level of energy expenditure; play, toy and sports preference; clothing preference; maternalism and maternal play; career ambition; body image; and the nature of the perceptual erotic arousal. I cannot expand on these categories here, but on all points the genetically and iatrogenically androgenized hermaphrodites closely resemble each other and differ profoundly from the genetically determined *anhormonal* condition. Evidence is thus available that in the human, as in infrahuman primates and infraprimate mammals, the behavioural potential can be influenced by the chemical composition of the environment of the embryo during critical periods in its development. All these experiments and observations have a serious implication for our approach to, and our understanding of, human bisexuality.

CONCLUSIONS

Cross-taxa behavioural comparisons have revealed that bisexual patterns of behaviour occur repeatedly as a normal, biological variation in a wide range of mammalian forms including primates and Man. Experimental evidence is now accumulating which points to the existence of bisexual potentialities, perhaps as distinct systems, in the mammalian brain which can be influenced during critical periods in development, in a male or a female direction, by chemical, hormonal means. There is a direct analogy here with the bisexual potential of the somatic, genital apparatus. Although enormous gaps in our knowledge remain, this newer data suggests that psychosexual differentiation in primates and also in Man is under some form of chemical control.

We do not know as yet what these substances may be, but experiments with adult-type hormones provide a useful model. None of the foregoing need be interpreted to mean that individual life experiences and social factors have reduced importance, for this is certainly not the case, but they can now be thought of as operating upon a substrate already given a chemical bias during development.

We do not have to account, ethically, for variations in coat or skin colour, or for the fact that some animals eat herbs and others meat. For me, the ethical problem presented by bisexuality as a biological variation is not to account for it, but rather to account for its ferocious condemnation in almost all modern Western cultures and, although the position is changing rapidly, for the defamation of individuals in whom these patterns of behaviour are expressed. It would be crudely to misconstrue the foregoing, however, were it taken to imply that homosexual and bisexual behavioural patterns are never symptoms of psychological illness which, of course, they often are. But neither is it acceptable in these days of casuistical or "situation" ethics to expose those who are ill to moral condemnation.

REFERENCES

Altmann, S. A. (1962). A Field Study of the Sociobiology of Rhesus Monkeys. *Ann. N.Y. Acad. Sci.*, **102**, 388–435.

Barth, K. (1958). "Church Dogmatics". (Ed. Bromiley, G. W.). T. & T. Clark, Edinburgh, Scotland.

Ford, C. S. and Beach, F. A. (1951). "Patterns of Sexual Behaviour". Harper & Row, New York, U.S.A.

Goy, R. W. (1968). Organizing Effects of Androgen on the Behaviour of Rhesus Monkeys. *In* "Endocrinology and Human Behaviour". (Ed. Michael, R. P.), p. 12. Oxford University Press, England.

Money, J. and Anke Ehrhardt. (1968). Prenatal Hormone Exposure: Possible Effects on Behaviour in Man. *In* "Endocrinology and Human Behaviour". (Ed. Michael, R. P.), p. 32. Oxford University Press, England.

Michael, R. P. (1968). Gonadal Hormones and the Control of Primate Behaviour. *In* "Endocrinology and Human Behaviour". (Ed. Michael, R. P.), p. 69. Oxford University Press, England.

Roy, R. and D. (1968). "Honest Sex". The New American Library, Inc., U.S.A.

The Problem of Abortion

MALCOLM POTTS

Department of Anatomy,
University of Cambridge, England

INTRODUCTION

Some systems of ethics are not founded on scientific observation, but any moral construct discussing abortion should take into account the facts of embryology, and one may be suspicious of views that are divorced from biological knowledge and reject those that are contradicted by it.

EMBRYOLOGY

For the first week of development the human embryo is invisible to the naked eye and the fertilized egg cleaves until a hollow sphere of cells, or blastocyst, is formed. The blastocyst can be kept alive in the uterus of another species; a sheep in a rabbit has proved successful and, no doubt, a human in a donkey is possible. Two or more blastocysts can be fused to make one individual, or one blastocyst divided to make several, and blastocysts that have been manipulated in this way can be placed in a host mother where they will develop to term. Such experiments raise interesting philosophical and theological questions because it is difficult to argue the legal rights of an object that can be turned into a chimera or separated into several identical units. The British Council of Churches has decided to equate conception with nidation (implantation) thereby excluding the first week of development from its consideration.

The egg, from the time of fertilization, is genetically unique but this fact must be seen against the richness of all biological processes and does not of itself warrant the immediate interest of society or of theologians. Every cell in the body has all the genetic information to make a new individual and botanists have been able to take a single cell from a root or leaf and grow a new plant without involving the germ cells in the process. It is possible that embryologists may be able to do the same for metazoan animals in the foreseeable future and it might, for example, be possible to take a single blood cell and develop a new individual, who would be an identical twin of the donor of the white cell but of a different generation. (There are 35×10^9 leucocytes in an adult man.)

Genetic diversity cannot be taken as the touchstone of ethical significance. During his lifetime a normal man will ejaculate 3000 times or
more, each specimen of semen contains 2—600 million sperm and every
sperm, as a result of the crossing over which takes place between homo-
logous chromosomes during the formation of the germ cells, is genetically unique. If a man fathered 20 children in his life-time he would use
only one part in one hundred thousand million of his potential genetic
diversity. The nocturnal emissions of a celibate man in one year provide
more than sufficient genetic information to replace the whole human
race without repeating the same individual.

In the days following implantation the embryo grows relatively fast
but it remains inappropriate to ascribe it any social or theological
significance. For much of the early part of pregnancy the placenta is
larger than the embryo proper and for the first two weeks there is
practically no true embryonic tissue. Except for very primitive communities it has not been the custom of civilized man to attribute social
rights or theological significance to the placenta. Between one in 1000
and one in 2000 fertilized eggs give rise to hydatidiform moles, which
are collections of placental tissue (trophoblast and mesenchyme) and
often totally lacking in any vestige of an embryo. They fall under the
series of objects for which Canon 748 of the Roman Catholic Church
prescribes conditional baptism, as monsters of unknown status. Nevertheless, it is very difficult, on strictly legal grounds, to distinguish a
hydatidiform mole from an embryo: it is the product of a fertilized egg
and it is genetically unique. Another pathological entity which cannot
be categorized either theologically or legally is a teratoma—a mass of
tissue, often containing recognizable hair, skin and nervous system and
even teeth. It contains some or all the elements of a human being but
lacks any overall pattern and arises spontaneously, usually in the
gonads. It is not associated with sexual intercourse, although chromosome studies show that it sometimes has a different sex from its host.
Teratomas are removed surgically like any other tumour, they are not
protected by Act of Parliament, they cannot inherit estate and they are
not baptized.

It seems impossible, or certainly very out of place, to extrapolate back
to the embryo the ethics which we apply to the newborn or the adult.
Conversely, it does not follow that the man who destroys an embryo
will also kill newborn babies. Abortion does not, as has been suggested,
"breach an important principle by suggesting that the deaf, blind and
maimed are disposable." There is no simple definition of what is human
and what non-human. There is no single event marking the beginning
of life, there is no Rubicon to be crossed during embryological develop-

ment upon which we can concentrate and say, "Before this moment we have an object as trivial as a nail-paring; after this time we have an individual human being to which we must reserve the full sanctity of human life". An ethical system founded on biology must begin by recognizing that reproduction is a continuum which can be traced back to the time when the primordial germ cells are first recognizable in the yolk sac endoderm (at about the 20th day after fertilization in man) and it is still incomplete when a grandmother baby-sits for her daughter's children. During this long process fertilization is an incident which is biologically important but so remote from the interests of society that the woman in whose body it occurs has no way of knowing what has happened.

ETHICS

The simplest and most satisfactory ethic on abortion is to avoid ascribing any legal or theological status to the embryo during the first two weeks of development; beyond this time the embryo becomes increasingly important and at viability (28 weeks) the fetus should have the same rights as a newborn child. During the first three months termination may be used widely, after that time it should be entered upon with increasing reluctance. Every decision on therapeutic abortion must be made *individually*, weighing all the factors concerned.

Honest human judgements, recognizing if necessary that they involve some degree of arbitrary decision, are much more likely to be sound and constructive than are moral verdicts passed in an atmosphere of false ill-founded confidence. After all, it was the Nazis who were so clear that abortion was immoral that they made it a capital crime: it was the philosophy that produced the concentration camps that also carried out the last European execution for abortion.

There has always been some recognition that an embryo has a different status from an adult or new-born and no ethical system has ever succeeded in imposing even a theoretical prohibition on *all* abortions. There is a well known complication of pregnancy when the embryo implants in some ectopic site, usually in the Fallopian tubes but sometimes elsewhere in the abdominal cavity. About one in 300 pregnancies are affected in this way and on very rare occasions the pregnancy can go to term: there may be half a dozen people alive in the whole world who were never in their mothers' wombs. However, all current textbooks of Roman Catholic ethics allow termination of pregnancy in the case of ectopic pregnancies. The sacrifice of the potential life of the fetus in the case of ectopic pregnancies is usually justified by recourse to the argument of double-effect (the doctor is said to treat the diseased tube and he does not intend to kill the embryo). But this sophistry should be rejected: every Catholic surgeon, if not every Catholic theologian, knows it is untrue and it is revealing that the Congregation of the Holy Office in 1902 outlawed the surgical treatment of ectopic pregnancies as "direct killing of the fetus". Today, no Pope would have the courage to re-state the principle because it would mean condemning thousands of Catholic mothers to death (the bleeding from ectopic pregnancies is nearly always fatal). Looked at in detail, even the most monolithic ethical defences have cracks and when it comes to abortion Roman Catholic theologians, as well as Humanists, have abandoned absolutes and chosen to make statistically based decisions.

AIDS TO JUDGEMENT

There are a number of signposts which help in arriving at rational, reliable and realistic conclusions on terminating a pregnancy. The biology of abortion must be understood. It may be either spontaneous or induced and an appraisal of the former is necessary in order to decide the validity of the latter.

Two things are important about spontaneous abortion: one that it is common and the other that it is biologically useful. It is difficult to establish the incidence of spontaneous abortion because there is a universal tendency to under-report pregnancy wastage, and because many abortions occur before a woman is properly aware she is pregnant. In addition, the epidemiology of spontaneous and induced abortion is similar for age and parity and many criminal abortions are passed off as natural miscarriages. These variables are least likely to be important among women who abandon contraceptive methods in order to have a planned baby and Tietze has found a 7% spontaneous abortion rate in one such group (although the sample may have been biased towards women of high fertility). In a prospective study of women in an Indian village 10·5% of known conceptions ended in spontaneous abortion, but some under-reporting was likely. Experienced obstetricians, taking careful histories in groups of several thousand patients, usually estimate a spontaneous abortion rate of 10–15%. In women over 35 having their fourth or subsequent pregnancy 20% abort spontaneously. The highest pregnancy wastage occurs very early in gestation and much of it before the first missed period. A significant proportion of germ cells are abnormal and incapable of fertilization. Hertig and Rock, who have collected most specimens of early human development, estimate that of the eggs which are fertilized 90% reach the blastocyst stage (6 days), 58% survive to implantation (7 days) and only 42% to the twelfth day.

There is a dramatic contrast between a wastage of 50 per cent or more at the beginning of development and a death rate of one or two in a thousand which occurs a month or so after delivery—although the intrauterine environment is more favourable than that of a suburban bedroom or council nursery. Observation suggests that the biological status of the embryo is fundamentally different from that of the established human being living free from his or her mother.

The biological value of abortion has only recently been recognized but once the significance of the natural process is understood it is much easier to construct a valid and creative system of ethics. Biological destruction takes two forms. One is ageing and death, with which we are all familar. However, few people appreciate that cell death and embryonic destruction are also an integral part of normal development. All biological systems must contain a homeostatic mechanism for eliminating mistakes. During the development of the brain, for every cell that differentiates into complex functioning neurone, three degenerate. If this spontaneous degeneration and cell death did not occur the brain would be a formless tumour incapable of activity.

Many spontaneous abortions are grossly abnormal. The most accurate statistics come from the analysis of chromosomes. Among 227 unselected spontaneous abortions Carr found 50 examples of chromosome anomalies. This is fifty times the rate of chromosome abnormalities found at term and, in 51 controls taken from induced abortions and ectopic pregnancies of comparable age, no abnormalities were detected. Kerr has shown that the number of chromosome abnormalities declines with the duration of gestation, demonstrating the way in which spontaneous abortion progressively eliminates the pathological. Many of the chromosomal abnormalities discovered in spontaneous abortions are of a severity unknown at birth. Mongolism is an example of trisomy (an extra chromosome) involving one of the smallest chromosomes. Many abortions have trisomies of very large chromosomes. Mongols survive because biologically their defects are trivial and most are not aborted spontaneously. When a known teratogen, such as the rubella virus, affects a population there is an increased incidence of spontaneous abortion and, again, it is the biologically less severe abnormalities which survive.

Congenital abnormalities are becoming a relatively more important cause of death and ill health. In 1900 the infant mortality rate was 154 per 1000 and congenital malformation accounted for 1 in 30 of deaths. By 1965 the infant mortality rate had fallen to 19 per 1000 and the deaths due to congenital abnormalities—which show little absolute change—accounted for 1 in 5 of these fatalities. If spontaneous abortion did not occur, life as we know it would be impossible. At present approximately 1 in 50 of the population is congenitally abnormal, but fortunately most defects are minor. If all the abnormal embryos that were conceived survived, then 1 in 10 to 1 in 5 of the population would be abnormal and most of the defects would be gross and incapacitating. It has been suggested that thalidomide was not teratological but prevented spontaneous abortion. The hypothesis appears to be unfounded, but there is no biological reason why a drug should not be discovered which would abolish spontaneous abortions. The way in which such a drug might be used could be made into an interesting test of the practicability of any system of ethics dealing with abortion.

No congenital disease is curable although some, like cleft palate, can be repaired and others, like phenylketonuria, can be ameliorated. Some congenital defects are unpredictable but many are subject to the normal laws of inheritance. Achondroplasia, Huntington's chorea and osteogenesis imperfecta are examples of dominant conditions where, on average, half the children of an affected parent will have the disease. Certain of the muscular dystrophies and some metabolic defects, cystic fibrosis of the pancreas and amaurotic family idiocy are examples of recessive conditions in which both parents must carry the defective gene and the chance of a child manifesting the disease is one in four. Other conditions, such as haemophilia, are X-linked, so that boys born to a mother with the trait have a one in two chance of inheriting the disease and daughters a similar chance of becoming carriers. A number of conditions, such as anencephaly or congenital heart disease, have a complex pattern of inheritance but the empirical risk of having another affected child when one has been born varies from 1 in 30 to 1 in 50. The risk involved with teratological agents can also be calculated. In the case of rubella contracted before the twelfth week 7% of babies will have heart disease, 5·5% cataract and 2·5% deafness. Thalidomide is thought to have affected 20% of embryos when the mother took the drug between four and eight weeks of gestation. When the maternal organism rejects a pregnancy, or where there is a surgical interruption on eugenic grounds, then there is significant risk of sacrificing a potentially normal embryo. It is unfortunate, but not biologically anachronistic, to destroy normal embryos in order to prevent abnormalities. As is sometimes the case medicine may soon improve on nature and it may be possible to take samples from the extraembryonic membranes early in pregnancy in order to predict the likelihood of certain forms of congenital defect with greater certainty. This will reduce, but not remove the ethical dilemma; however, the problem only appears to be insurmountable if we perform the intellectual confidence trick of equating an embryo with a newborn baby. If there is a risk of defect and the mother is willing to start the pregnancy again then it is usually reasonable to perform a surgical abortion. The best protection an embryo has is to be inside a woman. The innate desire to continue with the pregnancy is usually more forceful than the theories constructed by man. To perform an abortion early in pregnancy may be creative of new life later, because a defective child can very easily absorb all a woman's capacity for motherhood and prove a barrier to further pregnancies. In a survey of 120 mothers with children having severe neurological defects, one third did not wish to have any more children and a further one fifth were very cautious about the possibility of another baby.

A useful biological guide to the status of the embryo is the development of the nervous system. The functioning brain contains many thousands of millions of complex neurones. The brain of the embryo, at the time most abortions are done, weighs one or two grammes and is physiologically very different from that of the newborn child or even the 16-week fetus. In defining death doctors are beginning to use the functioning of the nervous system as their main criterion and it may be that similar guide lines will appear in relation to the problem of abortion.

The Wider Problem

Most medical practitioners support termination for eugenic reasons and, more important, women themselves are overwhelmingly in favour of abortion on this ground. However, the very great majority of induced abortions are performed on social and humanitarian grounds. Do these constitute a licit, ethical extension of the arguments that have been applied to abortion for possible fetal abnormality? Does abortion on social grounds raise dangers, so that society needs to build protective barriers? If we accept that development is a continuous process are we left floundering unable to distinguish between abortion, infanticide and murder? If termination at 10 weeks, why not at 28? Are we on the Gadarene slope to euthansia, murder and genocide?

Firstly, there is the observational fact that many women have induced abortions, but few commit infanticide and murder by women is practically unknown. Women do not regard abortion in the same way as they do stillbirth or the loss of an infant, there is no mourning when a late period arrives or any attempt to baptize the menses, although there is a reasonable probability that an embryo may have been lost. Women do not equate abortion with murder but rather rally round to help one another. Emotive talk of the "unborn child" usually involves, quite literally, magnifying the facts. Perhaps complex defences have been built in the past to deter an army that never existed. Secondly, the credibility gap between practice and teaching in many ethical systems is so wide that even the most cautious moral thinker may be led to doubt their validity. The Roman Catholic prohibition against induced abortion is as far reaching as any, but many Catholic communities have a very high incidence of artificial termination of pregnancy. Exact figures for legal abortion are available for Poland, which despite its imposed Communist government remains devoutly Catholic and the sins of abortion are preached with monotonous regularity from the Sunday pulpit. In 1964, 34 abortions were recorded for every 100 live births and in addition some criminal unregistered legal abortions took place. In Colombia, which is representative of the most conservative wing of the Latin American Catholic Church, induced abortion is so frequent that it constitutes the commonest cause of death among women aged 15 to 35 and the consequences of illegal abortion account for 44% of all female hospital admissions. In France and Italy there is the rare combination of a strict anti-abortion penal code and a police force which, at least some of the time, tries to enforce the law on this subject. Nevertheless, criminal abortions run at a very high rate. In Northern Italy (Piedmont) the birth rate is almost exactly equal to that for Hungary (1965: 13·4 and 13·1 respectively) and the marriage rate and population structure is comparable in the two countries. In Hungary, unlike Italy, contraceptives are legally available but there remain 135 legal abortions for every 100 live births and it seems likely that a similar pattern obtains in Northern Italy.

In England the abortion rate is lower than in many countries. The National Opinion Poll in 1966 computed 40,000 induced abortions a year and, while there is good evidence that questionnaires underestimate the true rate, it is improbable that induced abortions exceed 1 in 10 or 1 in 8 live births. In the same National Opinion Poll survey, Catholics reported slightly more abortions than Protestants.

To a scientist, attempting to relate observed facts, the only immediate connection between established ethics and abortion is one of almost complete inversion: in many cases, the more strict the taboos against induced abortion, the more likely are the followers of the system to engage in the practice. Perhaps the most important reason for the divorce between practice and theory is that the majority of ethical thought is founded on a particular interpretation of Christian theology. This influence is not only powerful wherever the Church holds sway, but it has given rise to much legislation and, as European laws have formed the basis of the penal code in many extra-European countries (such as India), it has become the accepted position for much of the world. Japan and China are notable exceptions.

Until the beginning of the nineteenth century theology, the law and the facts of biology were in reasonable harmony. The ordinary facts of life lead to an epigenetic view of development: a woman knows she is pregnant when her periods cease, some time later (at about 16 or 17 weeks) she is aware of fetal movements and anything that is aborted during the first trimester of pregnancy is not obviously human. For much of its history the ethical teaching of the Church gave implicit approval to this concept of increasing complexity and the infusion of the soul was considered to take place some time after conception. The theological doctrine of Creationism—every soul being the individual creation of God—became the accepted teaching of the Mediaeval Church and a distinction was made between the *embryo animatus* and *inanimatus*. The common law, taking its lead from theology, did not consider termination before "quickening" illegal. In 1803 the common law concerning abortion was put on a statutory footing but the punishment for criminal abortion remained much less if abortion took place before rather than after "quickening".

By a sad irony, Christian ethics became most strict and arbitrary on the topic of abortion at about the time that observational embryology began. The mammalian ovum was discovered in 1827 and the single-cell human ovum was not observed until 1930. Much knowledge of early embryology was discovered after good sectioning and staining techniques for microscopy were introduced towards the end of the nineteenth century and even today there are only a limited number of specimens from the first two weeks of human development. It is significant, then, that it was in 1861 that the English Parliament passed the Offences against the Person Act, section 58 of which made abortion at *any* time a crime punishable by a maximum penalty of life imprisonment. The 1861 Act remains in force although an exception for therapeutic abortion is possible under the 1967 Abortion Act. Likewise it was in 1869 that the Roman Catholic Church modified its previous teaching and invoked excommunication for anyone causing an abortion—however early in pregnancy, although at this time there was no factual knowledge whatsoever concerning the first few weeks of human development. The problem of the entry of the soul was shelved and today most Catholic apologists shy away from debating the time of baptism, basing their arguments instead either on an appeal to the right to live or on the particular genetic structure of the fertilized egg.

DIFFERENT SOLUTIONS

There happen to be some "control" and "experimental" situations which reveal the effects of imposing different ethical systems upon comparable communities. In Hungary, since 1956, abortion has been available "if the applicant insists on the interruption of pregnancy". This is the mirror image of many countries, such as Italy or France, where society insists that a woman keeps her pregnancy even if it endangers her own life. However there is no evidence to suggest that this situation has made family life any less stable in Hungary than in Italy. The number of first and second born children in Hungary is unchanged since the liberal laws were passed, but the number of women having their third or subsequent baby has fallen dramatically. Some indices of social health improve with liberalizing laws, for example, in Czechoslovakia (which also has liberal abortion laws) the incidence of illegitimate pregnancies has fallen in recent years, while in all western European nations it has been rising. The ethically most revealing statistic is found in Poland, where a very restrictive pre-war penal code was replaced by a liberal post-war legislation and the number of cases of infanticide known to the police fell from around the 1000 mark in the 1930s to 20 to 50 in recent years. It may be concluded that not only are social defences against the imagined evils of abortion unnecessary, but the host on the other side may actually be allies in the defence of social health.

NEW PROBLEMS

Biology gives new insights into the old problem of abortion and it provides a number of pointers which go some way towards solving a difficult problem. At the same time the assistance given is two edged, because it raises a fresh ethical problem. Doctors transfuse when there has been a haemorrhage, splint a bone that has been broken, tranquilize the excited, excite the morose, give insulin when the body's sources fail; are they in error to *fail* to terminate a pregnancy when there is evidence of fetal abnormality? Is this duty comparable to the physician's other obligations to carry out his healing role? Moreover the problem extends beyond the physical. Forsmann, in a follow-up of women refused termination in the city of Gottenborg, has shown that the children born to these women are at a social disadvantage. Compared with a control group of similar social background, sex and age, the "unwanted" children had more attendances at psychiatric clinics, more prosecutions for delinquency and drunken misconduct than their controls. In turn, the controls had spent longer at school and a higher percentage proceeded to a university education. The children whose mothers had sought abortions married at an earlier age than their controls, had more children and, 21 or more years later, appear to be making less stable marriages themselves.

It is sometimes difficult to decide on terminating a pregnancy but the responsibility to refuse a request to induce an abortion is also a grave one.

The Ethics of Organ Transplantation

M. F. A. WOODRUFF

*Department of Surgical Science, University of Edinburgh,
Edinburgh, Scotland*

Some knowledge of the biological basis of organ transplantation is required before one can discuss sensibly the ethical problems. Let me therefore begin by giving some background information.

Some people, as we all know, die of generalized disease; others live to a ripe old age and appear simply to wear out, rather like Oliver Wendell Holmes' "Wonderful One-Hoss Shay". But many people, like more ordinary mechanical contrivances, break down because of the failure of some particular part. This failure may result in little more than a certain amount of inconvenience, but on the other hand it may cause serious disability or, when a vital organ is affected, may threaten the patient's life.

Sometimes the loss or failure of a part can be compensated for either by some other part assuming an additional load, or, in the special case of an endocrine gland, by the patient being given the appropriate hormone. In other cases the question arises of replacing the defective part by either a mechanical appliance or a transplant, though of course whether or not this is indicated will depend on the severity of the patient's disability, the inconvenience and risk of the procedure, and the degree of benefit which can reasonably be expected.

The methods of replacement which are available, or which are likely to become available in the not too distant future, are as follows:

Mechanical appliances

    Prostheses

        Removable

        Built in

    Artificial organs

        Temporarily connected to patient

        Built in

Transplants

    Autotransplants

    Homotransplants

        From living donors

        From cadavers

    Heterotransplants

Dentures are a familiar form of removable prosthesis. Built-in prostheses are used in orthopaedic surgery, for example to replace the head of the femur, and in vascular surgery to replace diseased or injured arteries.

Artificial organs which are temporarily connected to a patient are exemplified by the heart-lung machine which is used to permit arrest of the heart during cardiac operations of various kinds, and the present-day type of artificial kidney used in the procedure known as haemodialysis. This was originally used only for "acute dialysis", i.e. the temporary treatment of patients whose own kidneys were thought to have some chance of recovering within a few days or weeks, but it is now used also for "chronic dialysis", i.e. repeated treatment at intervals of a few days of patients whose own kidneys are known to be irretrievably damaged.

Artificial organs which can be permanently built into a patient are not yet available, but I surmise that the next decade will see the development of an artificial heart.

Autotransplants are pieces of tissue or organs transplanted from one part of the patient's body to another. Autotransplants of skin, cartilage, tendon and bone are widely used in plastic and orthopaedic surgery, and for a variety of technical reasons it is sometimes necessary to move organs from one place to another, but this type of procedure is clearly not going to help the patient whose life is threatened by irreversible failure of some vital organ.

Homotransplants (nowadays often termed allotransplants) are transplants from some other person (or in animal experiments from one animal to another of the same species). As a general rule they survive for a few days or weeks but are then destroyed as the result of an immunological reaction which they evoke in the recipient. Some homo-transplants are therapeutically useful even though they do not survive very long, either because they tide the patient over a temporary crisis, as in blood transfusion, or because, as in transplants of bone, they provide a scaffolding which facilitates regeneration of the patient's own tissue. Usually, however, success depends on the transplant not only surviving but maintaining a satisfactory level of functional activity, and it is therefore fortunate that there are exceptions to the rule that homotransplants are rapidly destroyed, notably when the tissue transplanted is avascular like the cornea, when the donor and recipient are "histocompatible", and when the recipient's reaction to the transplant has been abolished or weakened by some immuno-suppressive therapeutic procedure.

Complete histocompatibility occurs when the donor and recipient are identical twins; with randomly chosen donors there is a wide range of degrees of compatibility. The development of tests for measuring the degree of compatibility prior to transplantation is an important objective of research, because it is more difficult to prevent rejection when there is gross incompatibility, and there has been encouraging progress in this field.

The organ which has been most frequently transplanted clinically is of course the kidney, and a recent report of the Human Kidney Transplant Registry contains an analysis of 1741 such operations collected from 89 centres in some 22 different countries. The results for the past two years show that kidneys from related living donors have a one-year survival of 75% and a two-year survival of 67%, while kidneys from cadavers have a one-year survival of 45% and a two-year survival of 38%. Many patients are alive after periods much greater than two years; our own series, for example, includes a young man who is alive and well more than six years after receiving a kidney from his father.

Attempts are sometimes made to compare the results of renal transplantation and dialysis as if these were alternative methods of treatment; they are, however, complementary. Dialysis is essential in preparing patients for transplantation in the first instance, and also for re-transplantation if the first transplant is rejected; it is also required temporarily after operation if, as is often the case when cadaver donors are used, the transplant does not immediately begin to function, since given this support excellent function may develop even in transplants which have not produced any urine for as long as three weeks. Dialysis alone means that the patient is machine-dependent for the rest of his life and some find this unbearable; moreover the best patients on dialysis are not nearly as fit as those with the most successful transplants. Finally, and this I think is decisive, inter-mittent dialysis and transplantation fail for different reasons; the former because available "shunt sites" (at which the patient's blood vessels are connected to the machine) become exhausted; the latter because of transplant rejection or some complication resulting from the immunosuppression. In consequence, by using both procedures the patient's expected length of survival can be increased, and should theoretically approach the sum of the expected survivals for each procedure if used alone.

Attempts at transplantation of the liver have been made in several clinics during the past five years. The early patients all died but four of six children who received orthotopic liver transplants in Starzl's clinic were alive when last reported (Starzl, 1968) after periods ranging from 1 to 7 months. One adult patient of Calne's made good progress for nearly three months but has recently been reported to have died.

Following the experimental work of Shumway *et al.* (1967) and Cleveland and Lower (1967) on orthotopic heart transplantation in the dog, Barnard (1967) and his collaborators performed the first human heart transplant in December, 1967. The patient lived for 18 days; their second patient, however, is alive eight months after transplantation. A few weeks ago, some 26 operations had been performed; many of the patients were dead but some were still alive. Today, according to the daily press, this number has increased to over 50. There have been five reported cases of transplantation of the lung, but all the recipients have died from 7 to 18 days after the operation, mainly from infection.

Transplantation of the liver, and to a less extent the heart, presents special technical difficulties but these are not insurmountable; the immunological barrier is probably no greater than in the case of the kidney and may well be less, especially with liver transplants. Why then are the results so poor in comparison with those of transplantation of the kidney? There are many contributory factors but the decisive one is that there is as yet no artificial liver or heart comparable to the artificial kidney which can compensate over a period of days or weeks for loss of function of the corresponding natural organ. Since the patient's own heart or liver is generally removed and replaced by the transplant this must develop good function immediately if the patient is to survive. In the case of the kidney, before chronic dialysis became available this was achieved by relying on living donors, but obviously hearts and livers for transplantation can only come from cadavers.

Heterotransplants are transplants from an animal to man (or experimentally between animals of different species). The problem of preventing rejection is even more formidable than in the case of homotransplants; recent work has shown, however, that it is soluble in respect of certain tissues and species combinations so that the possibility of replacing human organs with organs from animals no longer seems as remote as it did a few years ago. If this could be done with organs from some common domestic or farm animal it would be of great practical importance; if, however, the only possible donors were higher apes the supply problem might well prove to be even more difficult than the immunological one.

So much for the biological facts. Turning now to the ethical issues let me begin with the proposition, which I think all medical practitioners would accept, that a doctor's primary responsibility is to his patient; to try to preserve life, to restore physical and mental health, and to relieve suffering. At first sight this seems straightforward enough, but in practice it is often difficult to decide on the right course of action to pursue, partly because these various objectives are not always mutually compatible, and partly because there is sometimes no established effective treatment for the condition from which the patient is suffering. What degree of suffering should we be prepared to inflict on our patients in return for a faint hope of saving life? When, if ever, should we be prepared to try a new form of treatment which has never been tried before? Moreover, despite its paramount importance the doctor's duty to his patient is not his only responsibility; there are many other people to be considered, including people who may be affected directly or indirectly by the patient's illness, people who have, or at some future time are going to develop, the same disease as the patient, and, of special importance in relation to our present discussion, transplant donors and potential donors, and their close relatives.

From the recipient's point of view the expected results of transplantation have to be considered in relation to the probable outcome if either nothing is done or the patient is treated in some other way. Some distinguished people have expressed the fear that transplantation may prolong life unduly; others appear to base their objection to the procedure on the ground that it does not make the recipient live for ever. A more reasonable criterion of complete success would be that the operation restored to the patient the life expectancy of a normal person of the same age and sex; this however is an ideal at which to aim, and much more limited success after transplantation, and many other types of medical and surgical treatment, is often of great value to a patient.

I have no personal experience of transplantation of the heart and liver but in the light of experience of renal transplantation extending over eight years I believe that it is proper, if a kidney is available, to offer transplantation to every patient on dialysis who has been adequately rehabilitated by this procedure and who does not suffer from any serious lesion of his distal urinary tract, and even, at least until the supply of dialysis facilities is equal to the demand, to exhort such patients to accept transplantation, provided the following conditions are fulfilled:

(1) The procedure can be carried out in a unit which has the knowledge and experience needed to cope with the manifold problems of donor selection and of patient management before, during and after operation, including the use of immunosuppressive agents.

(2) No other patient is accepted for dialysis in the recipient's place until the transplant is functioning satisfactorily.

(3) The dialysis programme has sufficient slack in it to allow of transplant recipients being taken back on to regular dialysis if this is considered necessary—on account of threatened graft rejection or drug toxicity—as it is likely to be at some time with the great majority of recipients of transplants from donors other than identical twins.

But what of the transplant donor? In my opinion it is right to allow a healthy individual of sound mind and stable personality who possesses two normal kidneys to donate one to a relative or possibly to a close friend who is suffering from irreversible renal failure provided that: (a) transplantation from a cadaver is not feasible, owing, for example, to shortage of supply or to special difficulty in maintaining the patient by dialysis before and after operation; (b) the general condition of the patient and the degree of donor-patient compatibility are considered satisfactory; (c) the probable result of the operation so far as the recipient is concerned, and the risk, immediate and remote, to the donor have been fully explained and understood. It goes without saying that the donation must be entirely voluntary; in particular there must be no threats or bribes, open or implied, and if it is felt that the prospective donor has been subjected to pressure and would like to withdraw his offer he should be at once rejected as unsuitable.

Discussion about the propriety of using organs from cadavers is often confused because of disagreement about what constitutes a cadaver. There are, I would suggest, really two questions to be considered here: What do we mean by death, and how can this condition be diagnosed? The first is a general question which properly concerns everyone; the second is technical and it is in my view the responsibility of the medical profession to answer it.

Death can of course be defined in various ways and compilers of dictionaries offer various suggestions. The Oxford English Dictionary gives, *inter alia*, "the final cessation of the vital functions of an animal or plant"; Larousse expresses the same idea more compactly as "cessation définitive de la vie", and goes on to draw a useful distinction between death and apparent death. Webster gives "the ending of *all* (my italics) vital functions without possibility of recovery either in animals or plants or any parts of them"; this is clearly related to the biological concept of cellular death and would seem to carry the implication that the vast majority of people who are buried are buried alive. A theologian may define death as the departure of the soul, but this would seem to pose an insoluble problem for those whose responsibility it is to draw up diagnostic criteria.

But if we must accept that the statement "X is dead" means different things to different people we need not stop there. Fortunately there is at least one common inference which the vast majority of ordinary men and women draw from such a statement, namely, that the time has come to dispose of X's body, normally by burial or cremation. Moreover it is clear that people as individuals and civilized societies look to doctors to say when this time has arrived and to give formal expression to their views by signing a death certificate.

If we adhere to this notion that a person is dead when and only when ordinary doctors would have no hesitation about signing a death certificate and ordinary people would have no qualms about disposing of the body, then the removal of organs from a cadaver for use as transplants does not to my mind pose any ethical problems, so long as known wishes of the deceased concerning the disposal of his body and its various parts are respected.

This leaves us, however, with another question, namely, whether organs obtained after death (in the above sense of the word) are likely to be useful as transplants. Many subjects are of course unsuitable as donors in consequence of the nature of their disease, or because their organs have suffered irreparable damage during the last few days or hours of life; when this is not the case, however, satisfactory kidney transplants can be obtained provided that they are removed from the body very soon after death—preferably within a matter of minutes and certainly in less than an hour. This brings an element of urgency to the diagnosis of death which has not existed hitherto, and may necessitate the development of new diagnostic criteria, but in my view this is a technical matter. It also implies that delay, such as now frequently results from the necessity of obtaining permission from relatives who may be difficult to contact, will inevitably result in the loss of potentially useful transplants. Here we come up against legal and logistic problems but again I do not see any insuperable ethical barrier. The real difficulty becomes apparent when we ask not whether some useful cadaver kidney transplants can be obtained but whether we can obtain an adequate number of such transplants, and also of transplants of other organs, commensurate with the demand. At present demand for kidney transplants greatly exceeds supply and for reasons discussed earlier the degree of urgency, and hence the supply difficulties, may be even greater with liver and heart transplants.

It has been suggested that these difficulties could be overcome by adopting a new definition of death based on total irreversible loss of cerebral function, which would be applicable to patients in which certain functions are maintained by extra-corporeal circulation and/or artificial respiration. These procedures are begun at a time when it seems possible that the patient may eventually recover, and I agree entirely that it is proper to switch off the machines if the time comes when an appropriately constituted group of doctors concludes in consultation that there is no possible hope of recovery because of total and irreversible loss of cerebral function. But this does not necessitate a new definition of death, and the case against such a change is in my view decisive. For in addition to the proposed new definition being inconsistent with the views of ordinary men and women, its acceptance would necessitate the introduction of a new term to indicate that a body could be buried, unless, of course, as Daube has pointed out, we are prepared to contemplate burying people while their hearts are still beating. No. Let us agree that there are circumstances in which the machines should be stopped; but let us adhere to the commonsense notion that while death will certainly ensue it does not take place the moment the switch is turned off.

The important question (and it is an ethical one) which remains is whether it is proper to remove organs for transplantation from a patient maintained artificially, after a decision has been made to stop the machinery but before he is dead in my old-fashioned sense of the word. Changing the definition would enable us to rephrase the question in a way which at first sight might appear more acceptable to some people, but it does not solve the problem.

REFERENCES

Barnard, C. N. (1967). *S. Afr. med. J.*, **41**, 1271.
Cleveland, R. J. and Lower, R. R. (1967). *Transplantation*, **5**, 904.
Starzl, T. E. (1968). *Antibiot. Chemother.* (Basel) **15**.
Shumway, N. E., Angell, W. W. and Wuerflein, R. D. (1967). *Transplantation*, **5**, 900.

Problems Raised by Developments in Genetics

C. A. CLARKE

Nuffield Unit of Medical Genetics, University of Liverpool, Liverpool, England

The contributions to this symposium have been clear, and fully comprehensible. Now this may, in part, be due to the excellence of the authors, but it is also accounted for by the fact that each paper concerns ethics—a subject in which we have all been trained from earliest childhood, and one that at the practical day-to-day level most of us find entirely easy to deal with.

Writing as a physician who actually has to cope with patients, I say that generalizations about ethical values are difficult, but when it comes to an individual patient there are usually combinations of factors which enable us readily to give a definite answer. This is helped because in our training we have had to learn to make up our minds one way or the other, even when the evidence is incomplete.

What medical men find more difficult is to understand the steps that have led up to many scientific discoveries. The contraceptive pill is a monumental piece of endocrine engineering; growing and counting chromosomes is a work of art; and many biochemical investigations are masterpieces of reasoned thinking. However, because most people do not understand endocrines, chromosomes or biochemistry at all—and newspapers need copy—ethical problems concerned with new discoveries are exaggerated out of all proportion to the likely consequences, and it is the Pope who steals the show rather than the scientists who designed the pill. Again, because good news is usually dull, journalists tend to speculate pessimistically rather than pay attention to the beneficial side of discoveries.

With this background in mind, let us consider a few medical genetic problems, and try to assess their ethical implications.

ABILITY TO CHOOSE THE SEX OF ONE'S CHILDREN

It is likely that it will soon be feasible to choose the sex of one's children, but it will probably mean artificial insemination using either X or Y sperm which have somehow been differentiated from one another. Parents might think this was a reasonable procedure if it

93

meant that their child was then able to inherit a title, for example, or a large amount of money; or if a child of a particular sex was seriously at risk for a genetic disorder. Otherwise it seems that most people would find artificial insemination distasteful, and I am sure that when young people marry and contemplate having children, the last things they consider are doctors, scientists or ethics. The experts, however, see a world of all male children, perpetual war, no mates, and a hopelessly upset economic system. I doubt this eventuality, and presumably any tendency to an upset in the sex ratio could easily be corrected by the General Medical Council!

THE ABILITY TO DETECT EARLY IN PREGNANCY (BY LOOKING AT AMNIOTIC CELLS) MONGOLS AND OTHER CHROMOSOMALLY ABNORMAL FOETUSES

This problem immediately raises the question of whether the abnormal foetus should be aborted—although in my view this is not a problem as such, because abortion should certainly be permitted (and even advised) unless the woman is particularly anxious to have the baby even if a mongol.

It would be interesting to hear the Roman Catholic view on this, and more hypothetically, on whether it would favour the preservation of life if all spontaneous abortions could be prevented (say by a new drug), even though this would entail an enormous increase in the number of children born mentally defective, since the great majority of chromosomally abnormal foetuses are spontaneously aborted.

THE ABILITY TO SEX THE FOETUS *in utero* IN RELATION TO X-LINKED GENETIC DISORDERS

It is now possible to detect by special tests most female carriers of haemophilia and the appalling Duchenne type of muscular dystrophy. The sons of such women have a fifty-fifty chance of being affected and now that sexing *in utero* is possible, abortion should be offered if the parents are unwilling to accept the high risk of having a male child. Conversely, if a male haemophiliac married, he might wish for a female child to be aborted, since these would all be carriers whereas his sons would all be normal. In my view this, too, would be ethical.

GENETIC ADVANCES IN TISSUE CULTURE

This subject can be divided into three parts; (*a*) hybrid cells; (*b*) the non-rejection of the fertilized egg; and (*c*) "clonal man". These have been grouped together because of correspondence for this paper arising from the B.B.C. television programme "Assault on Life" ("Towards Tomorrow", December 7, 1967).

(a) *Hybrid cells**

Cells from different parts of the body, either within or between species, can be made to fuse together. As a result, information can be obtained on the specificity of function, e.g. why a red blood cell makes only the protein haemoglobin and muscle cells only muscle protein even though both cells contain the genes for making both.

Similarly, virus-induced cancer cells can be fused with normal cells and as a result the virus can be detected, whereas it cannot be detected in malignant cells.

This is in my view a perfectly legitimate line of research of potential value to Man, and in particular to cancer studies.

An opposing point of view is exemplified by the reactions of one of the viewers of this television programme who misunderstood the work portrayed. "I watched with increasing horror and fear while scientists from the United States and Britain discussed and illustrated experiments taking place in laboratories in these countries to try and create different forms of life by combining the cells of different species . . . Are we to sit quietly by while the scientists produce the means to destroy the human species in the process of creating other forms of life? Can no one stop the scientists before it is too late?" (letter to *The Times*, December 14, 1967).

This seems to me to be unduly alarmist. The writer was ignoring the fact that scientists are usually responsible people; and that in any case hybrid animal cells are not hybrid animals.

(b) *The non-rejection of the fertilized egg*†

It is an accepted fact that organ transplantation is greatly hindered by the immune rejection response. In child-bearing, however, the womb appears protected in this respect. Experiments to clarify why this is so have been carried out by implanting fertilized eggs (from animals) into other tissues to try to discover why it is the uterus specifically which does not reject the foetus, even though this is half-foreign.

This gives rise to the ethical problem of whether this is a perfectly proper experiment. My view is that it is in animals, but that until more is known about the results, it would be unethical to take a fertilized human egg and implant it in the uterus or in any other tissue of an animal, e.g. a monkey.

---

* See Science Report, *The Times*, December 15 1967, and Harris & Watkins, 1965.
† See Science Report, *The Times*, December 15, 1967, and Kirby *et al.*, 1964.

(c) *"Clonal Man"**

It is now possible to take the nucleus out of the intestinal cell of a frog and implant it in an unfertilized frog's egg, the nucleus of which has been destroyed by a beam of radiation. The intestinal nucleus in the egg environment develops into a normal tadpole since the specialized cell contains all the necessary genetic information, although when in the intestine much of this is "switched off". Conceivably, therefore, it might be feasible to produce exact copies of desired individuals, e.g. Derby winners, first-class cricketers or other exceptional human beings.

If this ever happened, immortality would be assured and also, of course, members of the same clone could exchange organs with impunity.

Since mammalian eggs are extremely small, the technical difficulties in this cellular surgery would be enormous. It would be necessary to obtain an egg from a woman, kill its nucleus, implant a nucleus from, for example, an intestinal cell from someone else—and then re-implant the egg in a woman's uterus.

My view is that there would only be an ethical problem if "clonal man" were easy to produce.

It has been suggested (in a letter to *The Times*, December 14, 1967) that this technique might be used immorally to produce a subnormal race of willing domestic workers. Agreed, if they were subnormal; but why need they be?

"MAKING LIFE"

It has recently been discovered (see *Nature*, 1968) that a complete and biologically active viral (bacteriophage) chromosome can be synthesized *in vitro* by placing the appropriate bases and enzymes around a molecule of living DNA.

An extension of this work is the manufacture of an individual gene; if this can be made, it is intended to insert it into the chromosome of a bacteriophage which can then act as carrier to introduce the synthesized gene into a bacterial cell to see if it functions. If this ever became possible, replacing faulty DNA might become feasible and inherited disease avoided.

This would be very difficult in Man, but it would be eminently desirable in particular cases and I think the experiment itself is so elegant as to be equivalent to being ethical.

* See Taylor, 1968.

ETHICS IN CLINICAL TRIALS

The genetically determined disorder of Rh haemolytic diseases of the newborn can now usually be prevented by the giving of anti-Rh gammaglobulin after delivery (see Clarke, 1968).

During the course of the clinical trials, a sure sign of success was that the controls started to complain of being guinea-pigs. Experimental patients are not always the ones at risk.

A different problem in the same research has been whether it is ethical artificially to immunize Rh negative volunteer males with Rh positive cells in order to obtain the anti-Rh gammaglobulin. This is because there is a risk of introducing the virus of jaundice. With care, however, this is unlikely and we have felt covered by the fact that the men are volunteers and appreciate the risk.

It has been objected that it is impossible for a lay volunteer to understand the problem properly, but I do not think this is true. The volunteers, who are blood donors, are a very intelligent group of dedicated people, and if the full facts of the matter are explained to them, they can easily comprehend the risks and are very willing to take them if they feel they are really helping humanity.

AN ETHICAL PROBLEM RELATED TO CANCER PREVENTION

Some years ago, we (Howel Evans *et al.*, 1958) discovered two Liverpool families who had what is usually a quite harmless abnormality of the skin—tylosis (see Fig. 1)—which is inherited as an autosomal dominant.

However, in these particular families there was a most sinister association with cancer of the oesophagus (see Fig. 2) for part of one pedigree. We have estimated that, provided a tylotic individual lives long enough, there is a 95% chance of him or her developing the cancer, although the non-tylotic sibs are never affected. Therefore, we have had, for a number of years, a genetic marker for oesophageal cancer. The ethical problem has been how much to alert tylotic individuals in these families to the risk they run—i.e. to steer a course between the Scylla of being too casual and the Charybdis of engendering cancer-phobia. In this we have been highly unsuccessful, for all five of the patients who have since developed the cancer have died.

Cancer seems remote to people who feel well and (as in the relationship smoking and carcinoma of the bronchus) it is extremely difficult to present the risks in the right way.

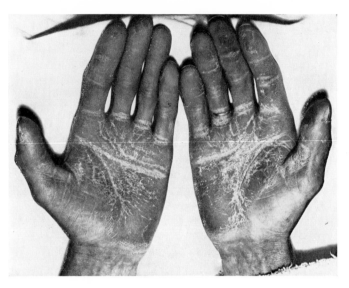

FIG. 1. Tylosis (syn. hyperkeratosis palmaris et plantaris) affecting the hands.
The soles are similarly affected.

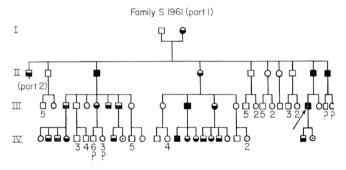

FIG. 2. Part of tylosis pedigree: □ ○ normal; ■ ● tylosis and cancer; ▱ ⬭ tylosis.

Conclusions

Advances in general come gradually and are usually unpredictable.
Therefore, speculation and too detailed planning should be avoided—
and bridges crossed only when they are encountered.

REFERENCES

Clarke, C. A. (1968). "Prevention of Rhesus Iso-immunization". *Lancet*, **ii**, 1.

Harris, H. and Watkins, J. F. (1965). "Hybrid Cells derived from Mouse and Man: Artificial Heterokaryons of Mammalian Cells from Different Species". *Nature*, **205**, 640.

Howel-Evans, W., McConnell, R. B., Clarke, C. A. and Sheppard, P. M. (1958). "Carcinoma of Oesophagus with Hyperkeratosis Palmaris et Plantaris (Tylosis). A Study of Two Families". *Quart. J. Med.*, **27**, 413.

Kirby, D. R. S., Billington, W. D., Bradbury, S. and Goldstein, D. J. (1964). "Antigen Barrier of the Mouse Placenta". *Nature*, **204**, 548.

(Anon). (1968). "Molecular Biology Comes of Age". *Nature*, **219**, 825.

Taylor, G. Rattray. (1968). "The Biological Time Bomb". Thames & Hudson, London, England.

Discussion

SLATER: In the matter of abortion, I should like to emphasize from my own experience in consulting with gynaecologists, the great importance of diagnosis as early as possible, and referral to the gynaecologist as soon as possible thereafter. It goes against the grain for the gynaecologist to terminate any embryonic life, and the more advanced the embryo the stronger this feeling becomes. Nurses feel about it just the same way. To carry out a hysterotomy for the removal of a recognizably human foetus becomes very repugnant. There is no reason why a diagnosis should not be made within a few weeks of the first missed menstrual period; and then, if abortion is called for, it could be done at such an early stage that the psychological trauma to all concerned would be minimal. As matters stand now, most terminations are carried out after long avoidable delays, only at the last moment before a hysterotomy becomes essential. These long delays themselves involve great strain and anxiety for the pregnant woman and her family.

POTTS: I agree completely. In addition, the risk of surgical complications associated with termination rises with the duration of pregnancy.

WALKER: There would appear to be a fallacy in the reasoning used by Dr. Potts. He attempted to justify induced abortion because abortion is known to be a spontaneous event. But death is also a naturally occurring event and this provides no justification for killing people. Spontaneous abortion is a means of ridding biological mistakes. (I am speaking teleologically quite intentionally). If we could be assured that induced abortion is only to be used in cases of irreversible congenital deformity, then, and only then, may there be some justification for performing the operation.

Dr. Potts has emphasized the continuity of the reproductive process which makes it difficult to decide when an embryo becomes an "individual". But the obvious break is surely the moment of fertilization. The post-fertilization product has the full chromosomal complement of an adult whereas the pre-fertilization gametes do not. This means that contraception must always be more desirable than abortion as a means of controlling reproduction.

POTTS: In answer to the first point, the biological mechanism which rejects abnormal embryos is rather imperfect and normal embryos are often aborted spontaneously. I believe it is ethical to risk destroying a few normal embryos in an effort to cut down the incidence of congenital abnormalities. In answer to the second point, I think it is self-evident that contraception is preferable to abortion and I have already dealt with the question of genetic individuality in my paper.

GOODHART: There is a practical point about an abortifacient pill that may become freely available. First of all, under the present law this could only be administered on the authority of two doctors, like any other treatment to terminate pregnancy, but of course there may be a move to alter the present Abortion Act. If so, we should remember that anything freely available is liable to misuse. Presumably it will be suitable for use only in the earlier stages of pregnancy, and in a prescribed dose; but whatever warnings are issued, they won't always be observed. With the example of Thalidomide before us, it would be wise to consider what might be the effects of taking 10 or 20 times the proper dose several weeks or months beyond the proper time. When such a pill is on sale to all and sundry, we shall find out the answer soon enough.

Dr. Potts has argued that human development is a continuous process, from the primordial germ cell to Granny baby-sitting, and that it is in principle impossible to define when a new human individual comes into existence. May I with great respect suggest that this is a view which is contradicted by biological knowledge? For there *is* a real discontinuity at fertilization, or to be pedantic at the "activation" of the ovum which is not necessarily always the same thing. This is the point after, but not before, which it becomes capable of completing its development without any further stimulus from outside. Once activated, the organism will carry on its development until it dies. That is what most of us would have called the moment of conception, however else the British Council of Churches may now have decided to define that word. But whatever we call it, it occurs at a specific point in time, after, but not before which, development can proceed; and that is a real discontinuity marking the coming into existence of a new biological organism. Whether this point has any special ethical significance may be a matter for debate, but arguments based on the premise that there isn't any biological discontinuity really won't do at all.

Surely the real ethical problem in abortion derives from the proposition that a human being, unlike any other living organism, has some rights to his or her own life. Not an absolute right of course, for most of us would agree that we can kill in self defence or in war, and perhaps when someone has forfeited his right to life through his own fault. More debatably, some would argue that killing a person who has freely chosen to die may be justified, and more debatably still this could be extended to defective infants or the hopelessly senile, unable to choose euthanasia, but whose own best interests may require them to die. But these are exceptions to a rule that a man has a right to his life, which we do not recognize for any non-human animal whose killing raises no ethical problems, at least if it is painlessly done. When a pregnancy is terminated, a living human organism, which had it not died would have grown into a man, is deliberately destroyed.

EBLING: I think Dr. Goodhart's fears about the dangers of an abortifacient being used in late pregnancy may be unfounded. If substances which interfere with the function of the corpus luteum, either directly or by suppressing pituitary secretion, could be utilized, they would have no effect after the first three months, because pregnancy is then maintained on progesterone secreted by the placenta.

DOWDESWELL: I feel that Dr. Potts has left it to intelligent thinking people to face the subject honestly, and at last from the woman's point of view. It is impossible for a man or even another woman to know the misery undergone by a woman forced to bear an unwanted child. I think it is quite wrong that she should have to endure the anguish of the pregnancy when all she may want is to devote her time to her husband, her children or her work. It is often forgotten that in addition to the wretched pre-natal period, once the child is born the mother has to look after it every day, year after year. Dr Potts stressed that what is *said* on this subject is often quite the opposite of what is thought. This may stem from teaching the young, in both home and school, that a woman is always pleased to have a baby. Set against the agonizing burden of an unwanted pregnancy, the "7-day blastocyst", the "sanctity of the foetus" and the "rights of the unborn child" become quite insignificant.

MASON: I want to oppose Dr. Goodhart's view that the interests of the unborn child and its mother are separate. I submit that they are the same. To lose a child is to lose part of oneself—the only comparable thing a man could experience would be the amputation of a limb. Nevertheless women have a deep, instinctive reluctance, used more or less wisely, according to their education and intelligence, to bring a baby into unfavourable circumstances of any kind and they would rather undergo abortions than persist with unwanted pregnancies. I would go so far as to advocate abortion on demand and that the decisions should be entirely feminine ones, subject only to medical, surgical and health circumstances being propitious.

There is another aspect of abortion, however, which I must emphasize as strongly as I can. I have just spent three months in Taiwan—an island smaller than Wales and even more mountainous, with a present population of fourteen millions and an expected population, with only marginal birth control, of twenty-two millions by the late nineteen eighties. Having experienced this order of density with eyes, ears and nose—particularly nose—I would say that any humane measure likely to help stem the increase of population should be sympathetically considered and urgently promulgated.

GOODHART: May I make a brief rejoinder to Mrs. Mason's point, that a woman has a right to do anything she pleases with her own body? Of course she does, we can all agree with that. But unfortunately more than a mother's own body is involved in procuring an abortion. Whatever anyone may feel to the contrary, it is incontrovertibly a biological fact that an embryo forms no part of its mother's body, right from the start. Whatever else it may be, it is a separate living human organism, inside and wholly dependent, in a sense even parasitic, upon its mother, but no more a part of her own body than a tapeworm would be.

POTTS: I am impressed by the comments of the two lady speakers. They confirm my view that the best protection for an embryo is to be inside the woman's uterus and that, when a woman seeks termin- ation, she has already gone through agony and requires sympathetic attention.

I remain unconvinced by Dr. Goodhart's arguments. If they hold true, then abortion must be equated with murder. There are inumerable examples of the way society fails to treat abortion as murder. I will provide only one rather personal example: namely, Dr. Goodhart is a colleague of mine, he knows I have performed legal abortions and we frequently meet in the course of our work, but I have never had the impression that *emotionally* he is committed to the point of view that I am a murderer.

TOWERS: Professor Clarke said that he could not resist putting his hypothetical question about the possible preservation of all spon- taneous abortions in order to elicit a Catholic view. I would find it easy to resist making this reply, but feel in some way bound, or ethically obliged, to make the attempt. I regard myself as a Reasonably Intelligent Educated Briton (to use a happy phrase coined by Professor Clarke), who by fortune happened to be born into a Catholic family and who has ever since managed to maintain his links with the church. At times the ties become a little strained, and sometimes rather tenuous, but nevertheless I speak from within it. The view of the church that we were given earlier has always, for those of us within it, been something of a myth, because we know from experience what a wide variety of opinion, what extremely active discussion and

what good debate there is amongst its members. This evident truth
is becoming more widely recognized now in the glare of recent publi-
city.

I may not be a "typical" Catholic (I'm not sure what the phrase
means) but I do know a lot of Catholics who think in ways like me.
So perhaps I can give something of the "feel" of the likely Catholic
response to Professor Clarke's questions.

To take his second one first: if it became possible to prevent *all*
spontaneous abortions, would Catholics be in favour of this? I would
say "no", and would add that an important principle is involved here
—important for Medicine as well as for Morals. Nearly twenty years
ago the late Pope Pius XII gave clear advice that there is never an
obligation on doctors to use what he called "extraordinary means" to
preserve life. His advice shows that the recent hysterical public out-
burst against the Neasden directive concerning patients who were "not
to be resuscitated" had nothing that was characteristically "Catholic"
about it. Actually what the church insists on is not simply respect for
life but also respect for death. A recent international conference I
attended on "Experimentation on Human Beings" heard a moving
plea from a non-catholic American doctor that patients should be
guaranteed the right to die in peace—which isn't always easy to
achieve these days in the technological palaces that some of our
hospitals have become.

As to Professor Clarke's first question about automatic abortion for,
say, a foetus that is discovered to be a case of mongolism, I would say
that this decision would rest on one's general attitude to mentally
defective members of the community. If society believes that they
should not be tolerated, then society will decide to destroy them, either
before birth or after. The real Catholic concern, as I understand it, is not
one for that mythical thing "the soul", but involves primarily a respect
for all creatures and especially human ones; Catholics would not tolerate,
in my view, such destructive practices as here envisaged. Catholics are
much concerned with respect for nature. A very interesting change is
coming over the thinking of theologians on these matters as they
recognize what is second nature to biologists, that nature is not a
static affair but is continually evolving, and that man is part of this
evolutionary process. We live not in a cosmos but in a cosmogenesis,
and the Catholic respect and concern for man is now being increasingly
extended to the rest of creation. This ties in very closely with Dr.
Fraser Darling's position in his paper (p. 117). I would suggest that
scientists should not despise the Catholic view, because we may in
time come to rely on it. The fact that we are currently living in a

permissive society certainly makes the church today look restrictive and repressive. But we should remember that it was not so long ago that a puritan society condemned the church for being altogether too liberal, in allowing, for instance, "wicked" things like dancing and drinking on Sundays. It is naïve to think that our permissive culture will last for ever—already amongst the young one can see signs of a returning moral, if not religious, puritanism. The extreme *avant garde* of today may have cause to be grateful for support against excessive puritanism, which the church will give again as always in the past. I was grateful for the responsible paper of my friend and colleague Dr. Potts; he and I have had many discussions over the years, and if he has influenced my thinking on the ethics of abortion it may be that I have influenced his in return. It is only through free discussion that we can undertake responsible decision making. These exchanges of view, when carried out honestly, are the only way to achieve that "properly informed conscience" that Catholics talk about.

FRASER DARLING: What I would like to say may be a digression, yet as the discussion has gone this does seem relevant: I would suggest that over the subject of human sexual indulgence the Church and Behaviourism have fallen into the same pit from opposite directions, namely, the "animal" (*sic*) nature of it. Should we not realize that characters and expressions are flexible to evolutionary development, adding to their potential without loss of primary function? For example, the feathers of birds were primarily for insulation, then they developed into organs of flight and later into patterns of recognition and indicators of hormonal condition and behavioural intention. All these functions are sustained. Sexual expression by the human being is primarily a reproductive function, but it does not have to halt at that point in evolution. The ideals of human sexual love have long been with us, but rather as museum pieces because cultural, social and economic factors did not favour general evolution along that line. Now, with woman's emancipation and free choice in love, the accepted style, sexual love itself within the monogamic ideal, has the opportunity to reach to its spiritual function, especially now that science has given us a large measure of control over conception. Sexuality, instead of being an expression to be restrained between lovers, is rather one to be indulged to its fullest. When love is so developed there can be no promiscuity, as a close examination of the tale of Lancelot and Guinevere will make plain. Marriage, you will understand, has nothing whatever to do with the monogamic ideal and reality; the impingement of civil contract on the glory of love is regrettable.

SLATER: I should like to comment on Professor Woodruff's paper. I am a psychiatrist and currently the editor of the British Journal of Psychiatry. About two years ago I received a group of papers on the psychiatric problems connected with renal transplant surgery from the living human donor. These papers were accepted and eventually published. Since then I have thought more and more seriously about this work, and I have come to the conclusion now that, if I were offered similar papers today, I should reject them on the grounds that the whole procedure is very seriously unethical.

A basic principle of medical ethics is the ancient *primum non nocere* —before all other things thou shalt not do harm. What is the surgeon proposing to do to the kidney donor, who is his patient and stands in a professional relationship to him? He proposes to put his life at risk in a major operation in which he intends to maim him. There is no idea whatever of providing his patient with any medical benefit, but exactly the opposite, to do irreparable damage which may at any time become critical to his life. Each of us begins his life with a limited number of nephrons, with an available margin to stand the ravages of time. By old age thirty per cent or more of our functional kidney tissue has been eroded away. We have no idea of the magnitude of the effect of the operation on the donor's life expectation, but we can be quite sure that it is diminished. Perhaps, with only one kidney, a man's renal capacities will be wasted away much faster than in the intact individual. Is the potential donor warned of these eventualities? We can, I think, be reasonably sure that the danger and the damage he faces are not unduly stressed; because the surgeon is, in fact, not looking on the donor as a patient to be helped but simply as a walking kidney-bank.

Professor Woodruff's claim, that no donor is accepted as such if it is shown that he has been under any emotional pressure, will carry no conviction to a psychiatrist. The evidence of these pressures is not easily to be elicited and where other relatives have not sought to influence a man, he is quite capable of putting an unfair pressure on himself. It is all too easy to "blackmail" oneself into unwise action out of a mistaken sense of where one's duty lies.

The economics of transplant surgery should also be looked at from the ethical point of view. What we are doing is to cannibalize the new model to keep an old crock on the road. Quite clearly, this is not the way to tackle the problem of obsolescence. One sees the situation in all its absurdity in heart transplant work. This is an immensely difficult job, which makes enormous demands on the resources of the hospitals where it is carried out and so on the community. In 1966, 152,383 men and women in England and Wales died of arteriosclerotic and degenerative diseases of the heart. How many of these deaths could have been prevented by the provision of a new heart, and how many others were? Obviously, the motive of doing something to reduce cardiac invalidism does not enter the minds of the surgeons engaged in this work. Obviously, however perfectly the immunological problems are solved, and however sure the operation becomes, no worth-while contribution to the health of the community will be made in this way. This work is not done in a spirit of kindness, to bring aid to suffering humanity. It is high prestige work and is done out of motivations which, at their best, led to the conquest of Everest, but which in this context are those of hubris and vain glory.

The Right to Reproduce in an Overcrowded World

A. S. PARKES

Christ's College, Cambridge, England

We hear a great deal these days about the rights of man. Manifestos descend on us from a dozen quarters, national and international, religious, social, legal and political. The final authorized text of the Universal Declaration of Human Rights was issued by the United Nations in July 1967, and 1968 has been named as the International Year for Human Rights. The UN Declaration is a long and rambling document with a preamble divided into seven "whereas"-es, and thirty Articles with twenty-eight sub-Articles. It reminds one of Clemenceau's comment, at the 1919 Peace Conference, on President Wilson's Fourteen Points, that "the good God himself only had ten." Moreover, though well-intentioned, it is highly unrealistic and appears, like rioting students living on the taxpayer, to be more concerned with supposed rights than with clear obligations. Incidentally, we may note that the Declaration is being violated in some way or other in most, if not all, countries.

It is indeed a remarkable document. The only reference to reproduction is contained in Article 16, sub-Article 1: "Men and women of full age, without any limitation due to race, nationality or religion, have the right to marry and found a family". Taken at it its face value this clause amounts to a licence for unlimited reproduction by all and sundry for any reason from loving design to unlucky lust. There is not a word about the consequences for the community of unlimited reproduction by individuals; not a word of special consideration for women, who sexually and socially are far more in need of a charter than are men. All the Articles refer to the environment, mainly the political environment, and there is not a word about a right to a sound genetic make-up; or to be a wanted not an unwanted child; or to living space in the world. Nor is there a word about the individual's relative inability to choose the kind of person he would like to be—apart from genetic factors he has little or no opportunity of choosing the very early environmental influences which play a major part in moulding personality. Nor does the Declaration show any signs of recognizing that, whatever else he may be, man is biological material and subject to biological laws which we ignore at our peril, or that, as emphasized by Hudson Hoagland, the human brain was developed as a survival organ just as were claws and teeth and that in some ways, even in science and much more in politics, we are still not very far from the jungle, or that man's fantastic technical development has wildly outrun his wisdom in using it.

But of all omissions in the UN Declaration, the most glaring is the failure to enlarge on the right, or lack of it, to reproduce in an over-crowded world. And there can be no excuse for this—it is now 22 years since A. V. Hill in his Presidential address to the British Association for the Advancement of Science on the "Ethical Dilemma of Science", pertinently asked whether the rights of man included the right to un-limited reproduction. This question requires an answer in any current discussion of human rights, because of the unprecedented and acceler-ating growth of world population. The present total is thought to be about 3400 million and it is confidently expected to rush towards 7000 million by the end of the century, a little over 30 years away. This remarkable increase—present and prospective—is not because of any corresponding increase in human fertility, it is due to the work of the medical scientist, aided and abetted by the agricultural scientist, in keeping people, especially young people, alive; and the process continues apace. The effect is, of course, most marked in areas where the birth-rate is still high and the impact of medical science has been compara-tively recent, resulting in an astonishing increase in the proportion of young people, which in some parts of the world makes up one-half of the population. Two totally different and widely separated countries, Pakistan and Mexico, provide excellent examples of this state of affairs, but there are many others.

As biologists, we have here a classic example of the effect of relaxing one of the three main factors which in nature limit the growth of populations—food supply, disease and enemies. In nature also, the re-laxation of one of the limiting factors allows the population to increase until it bumps up against one of the other limiting factors or against the same factor again, perhaps in a different form. In the case of disease, the emphasis might shift from infective disease to organic disease or to the pathological, self-regulatory effects of overcrowding, or cultural patterns might emerge with population-limiting effects, but long before this stage was reached the world would be in uproar. Unless, therefore, we are to put back the clock of medical and agricultural science and rely again on infective disease and famine to control world population, or to decimate mankind with nuclear weapons, we must introduce conscious limitation of our numbers.

There can be little doubt as to where such limitation should start. To the Declaration of Human Rights I should add a Declaration of Human Obligations, one Article of which would run:

It is an obligation of men and women

(a) Not to produce unwanted children.

(b) Not to take a substantial risk of begetting a mentally or physically defective child.

(c) Not to produce children, because of irresponsibility or religious observance, merely as a by-product of sexual intercourse.

(d) To plan the number and spacing of births in the best interest of mother, child and the rest of the family.

(e) To give the best possible mental and physical environment to the child during its most formative years and to produce children, therefore, only in the course of an affectionate and stable relationship between man and woman.

(f) However convinced the individual may be of his or her superior qualities, not for this reason to produce children in numbers which, if equalled by everyone, would be demographically catastrophic.

Whatever their private performance may be, few would disagree publicly with Clauses (a) to (d) of this Declaration and we may hope that time will bring their acceptance in practice as well as in theory. Clause (e) is probably a counsel of perfection, and in any case it can be argued that many of those who have most influenced human history have had anything but happy childhoods. But all these clauses are still compatible with producing families far in excess of demographic ideals, and the real problem comes with Clause (f). Large families of the kind seen in Victorian times, which in spite of high child mortality quadrupled the population of this country in the nineteenth century, are now much less common, but they do occur. Where this happens with intelligent and knowledgeable people, one wonders about their background thoughts —are they inordinately fond of children, or are they debarred by their religion from contraception but not from intercourse? Alternatively, are they so convinced of their superior qualities and of the hereditary transmission of such qualities, that they feel it a duty to produce an exceptionally large family? And here we get into very difficult ground, both biologically and sociologically. There are, as Galton pointed out in his book "Hereditary Genius", well-known examples of exceptional talent appearing in generation after generation of a family, but there are more numerous examples of what may be called genetic flash-in-the-pans, and it seems to be accepted that the great reservoir of talent lies in the genetic pool held by ordinary people. Lest this be thought of as mere academic hair-splitting, let me hasten to say that in the light of the global population explosion and the ever shrinking proportion of the human race inhabiting this country, the question of quality versus quantity is a vitally important one. But there are enormous difficulties. Few people are good judges of their own abilities, fewer still can accurately assess their genetic value to the community. Intelligence tests give little indication of ability in any particular walk of life, and, if they did, ability is of little value without the personality and force of character to use it to the full. Evidently, therefore, only a very bold man says "I am superior material and I must have a lot of children even if it means, from the community point of view, that others must have fewer and must help pay for mine". And this brings us to the next point— what in the modern context is meant by a large family or a small one, and what is the relation between family size and population growth?

The current rate of growth of world population is about 2% a year, and simple calculations show that this rate cannot be maintained indefinitely because, even if food and other resources could be built up correspondingly, nuclear wars avoided, and existing and new diseases controlled, we should, quite simply, run out of living space. In the light of these considerations, what rate of population-growth might be acceptable? A strong case can be made for an all-out effort to stabilize world population at its present level. In many parts of the world this would cause in 40 or 50 years a large excess of old people compared with producers, but in the meantime it would offer some hope of raising the standard of living to an acceptable level in all countries. However, there is no hope of achieving this aim in the visible future, the most that can be hoped for is to slow down the rate of increase to below 1% per year.

The next question, of course, is as to what sizes of family do these rates of growth correspond. And let us start here with the very simple fact that if everyone got married and the average size of reared family was four, the population would double every generation interval, say every 25 years. No scientist needs to be told where a geometric progression of this kind leads. Lower down the scale, if the average size of a reared family was two, the population would sooner or later stabilize. What happens in between is shown by the following table adapted from Cox (1967).

These figures are based on the medical and social trends of the West but these are rapidly spreading to other parts of the world. It would seem, therefore, that an average family size of $2\frac{1}{2}$ would be the maximum compatible with a reasonable demographic target or, since

Average size of completed family per married couple	Rate of growth of population (% p.a.)
2	—
$2\frac{1}{2}$	0·75
3	1·5
$3\frac{1}{2}$	2·25
4	3·0

(From Cox, 1967)

children can only be produced to the nearest whole number, a 50—50 distribution of two and three children families.

Figures such as these show conclusively that in the context of the modern world men and women do not have the right to unlimited reproduction. An obvious corollary is that they do have the right to be informed about, and to practise, control of their fertility, which has a relatively enormous potential developed by evolution to combat the hazards of primitive life, and which is anachronistic in these days of medical and agricultural science. These ideas were well epitomized by the theme of the IPPF Conference held in Santiago, Chile, in 1967, "Planned Parenthood, a Duty and a Human Right". I have said something about the duty aspect. How about the right to control our fertility? The short answer is that the situation is far better than it was, but still not good enough. Interest in avoiding conception is probably as old as the realization that intercourse could lead to conception, but at various times and in many places it has been overwhelmed by social taboo and religious dogma, both, perhaps, enshrining the desire of leaders that their followers should outbreed others.

Our own country, though not as afflicted as some, has no reason to be proud of its record. A major eruption took place in 1877 when Charles Bradlaugh and Mrs. Besant reprinted a doctor's pamphlet on birth control and were brought before the Lord Chief Justice. They were accused of "unlawfully and wickedly devising and contriving . . . to invite and encourage subjects of the Queen to indecent, obscene, unnatural, and immoral practices and bring them to a state of wickedness, lewdness and debauchery." The charge was ultimately dismissed because of a technical fault in the indictment. It is hard to imagine that the defect was one of omission.

Some ten years later a doctor was struck off the Medical Register for publishing a sensible and useful little book called "The Wife's Handbook", which contained a chapter on "How to prevent conception when advised by the doctor". This, however, was only the beginning of trouble for the family planners. The great American pioneer Margaret

Sanger was imprisoned several times in the early 1920's for advocating birth control and I myself saw Marie Stopes, at one of her meetings about the same time, savagely heckled by what appeared to be otherwise peaceful and respectable people. Even as late as 1941, a learned judge—if that is the right adjective—based a judgement in a matrimonial case on his firm belief that contraception was not a matter of common knowledge—and this at a time when a survey showed that nearly 50% of newly married couples were using contraception. One effect of this taboo was that, with the honourable exception of J. R. Baker in Oxford, technical problems received little or no practical attention from biologists, and as a result, available methods of contraception remained technically archaic and aesthetically objectionable to many people.

Since World War II there has of course been a radical change in the situation. Contraception has emerged very much into the open, as a subject both for biological and medical research, and for public discussion. This change has arisen partly from the liberalizing of public opinion and partly from the recognition of the so-called population explosion. Partly, however, it has been due to the development of methods of contraception not contemporaneous with coitus, so that the "pill" and even the IUD have become subjects of conversation at times and in places when few people would feel that discussion of the cap and condom was appropriate.

This brings me to another point. I have said that the obligation to limit family size carried with it a right to be informed about and to practise fertility control by acceptable methods. But what methods? Present techniques for the most part are based on preventing fertilization of the egg. Without active intervention this means the use of the so-called rhythm method, based on avoiding coitus at the time when a fertilizable egg is likely to be present—the so-called natural method, though this is a strange description of avoiding intercourse at the time when nature meant it to take place. The difficulties and uncertainties of this method are well known.

Other methods of preventing fertilization of the egg depend on positive action and some, especially the Pincus-Rock oral contraception technique, are remarkably effective. All such methods, however, presuppose that intercourse is anticipated, and there is urgent need for a method acting retrospectively—picturesquely called by the Americans the "morning after" pill. There are signs that such a technique, demonstrated exactly 30 years ago on laboratory animals, is at last on the way for the human subject. But it does raise the question of what, in man, constitutes conception; here I would unhesitatingly say that it means not fertilization of the egg but implantation of the blastocyst in the uterus several days later. In other words, prevention of nidation, whether by destroying the fertilized egg or by preventing its implantation, is a legitimate method of contraception. Such a technique would be invaluable for dealing with situations arising from unexpected intercourse for which anticipatory forms of contraception are, of course, useless.

There remains the question of abortion, which is certainly a method of birth control, but is equally not a method of contraception. Here we may recall that last year, after a bitter Parliamentary battle in which every device of obstruction and filibuster was deployed by the opposition, a Private Member's Bill to liberalize the law reached the Statute Book. This was a notable victory for common sense and humanity, and one which I heartily applaud, but I should be sorry to see abortion become a routine method of birth control, except perhaps for a crash programme of population control in cases of dire necessity. On the contrary, it should be reserved for dealing with unforeseen medical situations or as a last resort when contraception has failed. I say this because induced abortion is biologically wasteful and, used routinely, it releases the man from responsibility for his actions, which in time should surely provoke women to revolt.

Technically and socially, therefore, things are on the move but we have still far to go. In this country, only a small percentage of women are known to be attending family planning clinics; the idea of biologically controlling fertility in men so that they can share the responsibility and the hazards, if any, with their womenfolk, is usually regarded as a joke; and legislation, even after last year's stride forward, does no more than permit Local Authorities to open clinics, which many still seem reluctant to do. On a wider scale, the Vatican still attempts to maintain its crumbling dogma on birth-control, not only over its own followers, but over the whole world—surely a sign of monumental arrogance and a gross violation of human rights. Again, the last State anti-contraception law in the U.S. was repealed only in 1966 long after Americans had started preaching birth-control around the world; Canada still has most stringent anti-contraception laws on the Statute Book, and so on.

But everywhere the opposition is in retreat or at least on the defensive, and there is ever-increasing recognition of the need to restrict human reproduction and of the right, therefore, of the individual to the necessary knowledge and facilities. Even the Catholic Church will sooner or later have to bow its stiff neck to the winds of change in matters of contraception, as it has often had to do in the past on other matters. Inevitably, this particular manifestation of the ecclesiastical urge to mortify the flesh will go the same way as the burning of heretics for the good of their souls and the castration of choir boys for the glory of God. In the meantime, those distressed and embarrassed by the recent Encyclical can perhaps take some consolation from the fact that, in contraception as in many other things, the sins of today are the virtues of tomorrow.

But where will our rights and duties take us? According to a recent estimate—guess might be a better word—coitus now results in pregnancy only once in 2,000 times, and with the urgent necessity for limiting population growth and the spread of contraception, this massive number will no doubt rise. At this rate we shall come to dissociate the idea of coitus from that of parenthood—a strange regression to the long period of human history when no connection between the two was recognized, and a strange development from more recent times when coitus was closely associated with at least the risk of pregnancy. And where will it all end? Will the intensive treatment of subfertility and the development of contraception cause high fertility to lose its survival value? Will the increase in the artifical feeding of infants threaten the survival value of the human breast, or at least of the capacity for lactation? Is the urge to frequent intercourse going to be the next thing to lose its survival value? Are we, in fact, heading to become a race of subfertile flat-chested women and unmanly men, able to procreate only with the aid of regular medical and psychiatric treatment? Maybe, but not in our time.

REFERENCE

Cox, P. R. (1967). The Demographic Characteristics of Britain Today and their Implications. *Eugen. Rev.* 59: 4, 222.

Man's Responsibility for the Environment

F. FRASER DARLING

Conservation Foundation, Washington, D.C., U.S.A.

Man is biologically an aristocrat. He has dominion over the creatures, the plant cover and the very landscape of his planet. Man, indeed, is privileged. Ecologically, he occupies the summits of food chains and pyramids. Man is the lord of the living manor and privilege is implicit in superiority.

I do not think aristocracy is a humanly conceived notion but an observable phenomenon. Beneath man are lesser lords on the summits of their own little pyramids, be they tiger or eagle, robin or mole, dragonfly or spider. The aristocratic ideal, however, is a conception of the human mind, very old, very beautiful, and a potential ecological factor of great significance in the world. Few races of men have quite failed to conceive this ideal though too little of it may have been practised either by groups, classes or individuals.

Briefly put, the ideal is expressed by saying that the aristocrat is the servant of his people. It involves the notion of restraint, what the Greeks meant in the word *"aidos"*. Superiority is accepted, not assumed in conceit, nor disclaimed in mock modesty; when superiority is known to its holder it is accepted humbly as a burden proudly carried.

I have no intention of giving myself to the wolves by discussing the virtue of the aristocratic ideal in its practice between man and man even if such a discussion would not be wholly irrelevant in relation to clean air and water as human rights, but I do take it as the basis of an ethic of responsible behaviour between man and his total environment. This includes all other living things, the landscape, air and water, and the various products of art in man's history, art being considered as an emanation of nature.

Civilization is itself a flower of evolution, one which man could not have achieved had he not learned to tap the immense stores of mineral and organic matter which the earlier planet had produced, and to modify the habitats in which he found himself. Immediately he ceased being an indigenous animal, recycling his products and wastes within his own habitat, he began to impoverish his world. Naturally, he could not see this straightaway, especially as he was still struggling to survive as a species. Nevertheless, there is evident in primitive

117

cultures a rudimentary sense of reciprocation to the environment or an identification as being part of the wholeness of it. When an Athabascan Indian asks the forgiveness of the bear he is about to hunt and kill because of his need, he is philosophically conscious and understanding of his own ecological situation which demands what the bear has to offer to his continued survival. His prayer is a beautiful example of restraint, no new-fangled hyper-sophisticated preciousness.

The earth has been rich enough to bear the strain of emergent civilization on its organic resources, and the gain is the beauty of the human mind, the glory of the human spirit. Yet all the time there has been a painfully conscious sorrow that the beauty and glory have been distilled from a mash of baser behaviour, emotions and physical evidence. Awe for nature and its expressions has, I believe, always been present, but the responses to that awe would make an interesting study of man facing and coping with his whole environment. Comparative religion is part of such a study and I think we should find that polytheism was an expression of man's sense of belonging to a whole of multiple checks and balances. An earth mother was functional and comforting even if terrible on occasion.

When certain wild crops could not be harvested and certain animals not be hunted until certain propitious dates, man was reaching to some scarcely articulate notion of conservation, to a facet of identity with other living things. The Dinka of the Bahr-el-Ghazal honours the giraffe calf born among his cattle by anointing it with cattle fat, and you will see even today how tame giraffes are in that part of the world. I have sat among a dozen Dinka men and women sprawled under one of their raised huts of boughs and thatch, and watched a tiny poisonous snake in the floor above us, weaving its way as confidently as a gecko. The little snake, an insect eater, was accepted; it was not outside the Dinka's world. The West Highlander still has in the back of his mind a half memory of Finoula's kindred; he will not kill a swan and is disturbed if some infidel does such a thing. This is more than mere taboo. The polytheistic attitude makes for a slow rate of change.

Monotheism was a powerful thrust forward for the human being, concentrating spiritual force, especially when man identified the image of God with his own—though he puts it the opposite way, that God created him in His own image. Now comes a process of dissociation with other living things and in the example of the Jews it extends to the notion of being God's chosen people. Here is enormous strength— at a cost usually unimagined and perhaps unseen until our own era. Western man, having adopted the Judaic-Christian religion, has not only banished all living things other than his own species from the partnership of God and himself, but has developed the convenient conviction that God created the rest of living things for the *use* and delectation of man. Orthodox religion may be tottering, but not this mental attitude; so-called rationality even strengthens it. My own plea for a preservation of a natural oakwood drew from a righteous and aggrieved timber merchant the expostulation "But it's ripe!"

Once life other than human has been relegated to the status of useful material, or material awaiting the discovery of usefulness to the human being, the return to an ethical system of thought relating to it is very difficult. I am not greatly moved when I hear supporters of the national park and nature reserve movement argue that living things have educational value, that the beauties of nature give pleasure to humanity, that they are of scientific value or of potential usefulness, and that we cannot afford to lose them. The essential attitude is not far in advance of that of the timber merchant.

Life exists in its own right and this we must acknowledge.

During my lifetime, philosophy, religion and science have come a long way nearer together. The philosophy of wholeness is grasped and accepted, and science now is less sure of any absolute distinction between living and non-living. "I was born a mineral and arose a plant. . . ." The truth of Zoroastrianism comes back to us, that we are all of one stuff, difference is only in degree, and God can be conceived as being in all and of all, the sublime and divine immanence.

If this is the point to which we have come, it is time for us to exercise the ideal of our aristocratic nature, to be the servant of the planet to which we were born and to which we are still bound. Neither life nor matter is to be squandered, but as yet the mercantile outlook remains paramount. If the cancerous growth of human population needs the destruction of more wilderness, then the human population must be indulged and more wilderness will be destroyed. I say cancerous growth because it is uncontrolled and out of control, resulting in the *barrios* of South American cities, the seething port cities of Asia where the food comes in—growth without form.

Pollution of the environment is a concomitant of over-population, but it is of two kinds, passive in that which no one can avoid, and positive in failing to act when the preventive process is known, either in sewage disposal or the control of industrial wastes. Here the aristocratic ideal is directly applicable between man and man. I think the National Coal Board has set an excellent example in its treatment of landscapes after open-cast coal extraction, and only the other day this body gave a subsidence area in Kent as a National Nature Reserve.

I spoke of man being a biological aristocrat living at the summits of ecological pyramids. The Scythians of the Kuban and the Ukraine, the Plains Indians of the prairies and peoples of deltas and marshes were comparatively few in number, living on high protein diets. As far as we can see, such ecological summit cultures are self-conserving of animal natural resources, but the descent from the aristocratic position in the change-over in land use to cereal production of wheat, maize and rice for sustenance and export has put such people or their invading successors in the position of shortening the food chain, going to plant food direct and finding wild animals either superfluous or a nuisance. The agriculturist feels an animosity to wild animals and they come more and more to be of some lower creation to be harried and slaughtered. The relinquishment of his ecologically aristocratic position has now landed man into the ultimate condition of rabbit and vole, without the merciful phenomenon of resorption of foetuses in times of excessive numbers. Yes, the potato will feed more mouths per acre than any other crop we have, but look at Van Gogh's "Potato Eaters", a striking social document, and read Salaman's *History and Social Influence of the Potato*. After that you can scarcely exclude dietary policy from ethics.

An ethical attitude towards animal life and towards landscape, pure air and clean water, has grown as our condition has deteriorated. The aristocratic ideal is there among the few but the real thrust forward towards conservation and care has come from realization of our growing plight and is not so much ethical as hygienic, concerned with survival. Even so, I think we are losing out. But such a complete pessimist as I sound to be must be a man of overweening conceit; in reality, we cannot take on the mantle of infallibility. Whatever we feel, we must act up to our convictions of the conservation notion, possibly putting back the catastrophe far enough that all men will have changed in heart. There are evidences in detail already in that the outlook for wild life in Africa is brighter than it was ten years ago, and this year at the International Union for Conservation of Nature research workers of five nations in whose hands the fate of polar bears is held, came together under a neutral chairman to discuss their work for the benefit of the bear. Even so, the inability of the powers to settle positively for conservation of the whale stocks of the world is a reproach to us. I think most of us do think of our behaviour towards the whales in the last forty years in direct ethical terms. The ethic of conservation is perhaps quite primitive, in that we recognize that we are not vegetarians and are not prepared to be so for some high-falutin' principle, but the stocks of animals must be treated with reverence near to veneration, not only because we need them and use them, but because they are worthy of respect in their own right as fellow members of the world community of living things. Such a view does not land us into any fantastic unreal world of Jainism. Aldo Leopold put it shortly over twenty years ago, "That land is a community is the basic concept of ecology, but that land is to be loved and respected is an extension of ethics." Land in Leopold's sense included the farmers' land and the whole terrain in which communities of living things lived; another short couple of sentences of his were, "We abuse land because we regard it as a commodity belonging to us. When we see land as a community to which we belong, we may begin to use it with love and respect."

Ecology as a science makes possible understanding as well as insight into what might be called the physiology of community. To use the ecosystem approach to study and assessment of land use and its problems is to make us readier to accept the ethical principles of conservation. An understanding of the intricacies of niche structure in biological communities causes us to hesitate in taking short cuts in practical thinking. We do not rush in with a spray gun at some apparent pest before we know what it does in its total community. Even the word pest is a doubtful one in the ecologist's vocabulary, for so often the pest is a consequence of earlier misdirected human activity. To instigate a chain reaction in ecological relations within a community on grounds of expedience is not only foolish but in my opinion unethical. We have done this in the past through ignorance, as in malaria control of the *Anopheles* mosquito, to find that we have brought other vectors out of the trees which are less easy to control. We did it with red mite control in British orchards. We could do it with tsetse control in Africa. The professed aim is always to solve an immediate problem or to provide urgently needed food for a not urgently needed human population. Sometimes it has been for the plain profit motive.

Ecologists facing social problems of biological equilibrium may be so far in the van in ethical thinking that they may be considered unrealistic. I think we need much discussion between agriculturists and the fringe industries with ecologists on the whole subject of ethical standards. Few of us can be happy with the degradation of living creatures now being suffered in the name of increased food production. Veal production by intensive methods, the de-beaking of hens and suchlike practices are the antithesis of the aristocratic ideal. It is doubtful whether such so-called farmers have really managed to lie to themselves (that purely human ability) that they are contributing to a worthy cause of food production for the masses. They are moved by the profit motive.

Orthodox religions of the Judaic-Christian phylum have failed us badly, historically in the Scriptures, philosophically in having split the community of life by the figment of soul as a human prerogative in association with God, and currently in their tardiness to face the consequences of uncontrolled human increase. Yet within the churches there are fine men with their eyes open and we should get in touch with them on the ideas of conservation. I tried this years ago with a Hebridean minister of hard-shell Presbyterian convictions and was told he did not concern himself with secular affairs; again, after drinking coffee with an Anglican bishop after a harvest festival service, I mooted the cogency of the conservation ethic at such a service and received the comment, "Candidly, I had never considered harvest thanksgiving in those terms." But it is time we tried again.

Finally, we should not lose sight of the fact that it is largely from Western man, deriving from the Judaic-Christian ethos, that the new ethic of responsibility for the environment is growing, but in so small a segment of power. Within it there is compassion as well as logic.

Ecologists are discoverers, not preachers, but how can they keep quiet in our present world? Nevertheless, let them not be mere expostulators, as so-called conservationists are apt to be. The ethic of conservation has grown up in a period of declining religious conviction, but I think this would be an inadmissible correlation. It has grown with our increasing straits, but not fast enough. As I implied at the outset, the social disciplines of subsistence cultures were often self-conserving of the habitat: a world which has so largely emerged from subsistence culture has tended to shed parts of these disciplines without understanding them and the habitat often breaks down along with the culture itself, and more so when technology is so powerful as to give false confidence. One might say this is digressing from ethics into social studies of an ecological character. All well and good, but there is a point in these processes at which ethical questions of behaviour and culture present themselves and worry us if we put them aside. At this moment we can evade them no longer. I, along with most of us, am seeking, seeking in the spirit of science, but with the feeling that science and religion cannot be far apart in such truth as may be vouchsafed to us.

As the dominant mammal on the face of the earth, as the clever one, the only one as far as we know capable of reflection and of accumulating knowledge, our duty is plain, to serve the lesser creation, to keep our world clean and pass on to posterity a record of which we shall not feel shame.

A Biologist's View of Biological Warfare

J. H. HUMPHREY

*National Institute for Medical Research,
Mill Hill, London, England*

The World War of 1914–18 was the first war of any size in which casualties due to enemy action outnumbered those due to disease. Until that time, in the Wars of the Greeks and Romans, the Crusades, the Hundred Years War, the Thirty Years War, the Crimean War and the Boer War—to take just a few episodes out of human race's recent war-like history— mankind's natural microbial enemies determined the outcome of far more battles than did his kings and generals. The point is forcibly put in Hans Zinnser's short book "Rats, Lice and History", which is good reading for biologists and should be compulsory for historians. Even the death roll in the slaughter of the first World War was dwarfed by the deaths due to the influenza pandemic which followed in its wake and swept away 25 million people, especially in those populations most disorganized and debilitated by the War and its aftermath. Until the advances in hygiene, sanitary engineering and preventive medicine of the last hundred, and especially the last fifty years, the increased ravages of disease were an accepted accompaniment of war—and there was little possibility of diverting them to assist one side against the other, even though attempts were not infrequently made to do so. Thus, in the important sense that its effects have (in general) been experienced in the past, biological warfare is not new. What is historically new is the possibility of living at peace—or of fighting wars—*without* infectious diseases playing a dominant role. Biological warfare would consist in attempting to reverse this. Although systematic studies of how to do so are known to be going on in the U.S.A. (whose Department of Defence is quite frank about them) and presumably elsewhere, no serious use of biological weapons in war has occurred so far. Consequently to discuss one's attitude to biological warfare as such is somewhat unrealistic, and I prefer to consider biological weapons, which represent preparation for biological warfare —whether or not they are intended to be used.

Let us start with a definition, which is hard to better, taken from a pamphlet on Effects of Biological Warfare Agents published in 1959 by the U.S. Department of Health, Education and Welfare. "Biological warfare is the intentional use of living organisms or their toxic products to cause death, disability or damage in man, animals or plants. The target is man, either by causing his sickness or death, or through limitation of his food supplies or other agricultural resources. Man must wage a continuous fight to defend himself, his animals, and his plants in competition with insects and micro-organisms. The object of biological warfare is to overcome these efforts by deliberately distributing large numbers of organisms of native or foreign origin, or their toxic products, taking full advantage of the ability to utilize more effective methods of dissemination and unusual portals of entry. Biological warfare has been aptly described as public health in reverse''. This is a blanket definition. Like the Geneva Protocol of 1925 it makes no distinction between lethal and non-lethal agents, nor between human and agricultural targets. In so far as microbial products, such as botulinum toxin, are inert, the definition even covers part of what might be thought to be chemical warfare; nevertheless it makes sense, in that the techniques required for manufacture and assessment are those of the biologist. For the purposes of this Symposium such a broad definition may suffice, and because it allows no exceptions it may even be the only kind of definition suitable for an international instrument banning the use of biological weapons. However, it should really only be accepted after a lot of hard thought about whether there is a valid distinction to be made between lethal and non-lethal agents, and between those aimed at man himself and at his resources. Before returning to this, it is as well to consider what are the special military features of biological weapons. These can be regarded under the headings of the claimed advantages and the likely disadvantages:

Claimed Advantages. The first is the enormous potential effectiveness per unit weight, which derives from the fact that microbes multiply in their hosts. (An extreme case, often cited, is infection of man with an estimated dose of 25 "Q" fever organisms, when inhaled as an aerosol of suitable particle size.) Others are cheapness to produce; difficulty in detection before infection has taken place, and (especially if the organisms have been introduced by an unwonted route) in identification after infection in time to apply specific therapy; ability to reach an enemy concealed or protected from conventional explosive weapons; avoidance of destruction of property and fixed installations. A final advantage claimed is that a non-lethal but temporarily completely incapacitating biological agent—such as might be Dengue fever introduced via the respiratory tract—could actually be an humane weapon by achieving the desired military effect without permanently maiming the enemy.

Probable Disadvantages. The disadvantages are twofold. The first are technical and reflect the difficulty of disseminating what are often very delicate microbes in a manner which preserves their viability and yet enables them to reach their target over a wide enough area, in sufficient concentration, and by a route which ensures effective penetration into the body. For practical purposes this means as an aerosol of particles 1–5 μm. Such problems are difficult, but in principle soluble—and may indeed, for all we know, already have been solved. The second are more strictly biological, and relate to the difficulty of predicting the attack rate, incubation period, mortality and subsequent spread in an exposed population. Although an intelligent guess could probably be made on the basis of animal experiments together with serological information about natural immunity of the target population, I doubt very much whether the degree of certainty which a military commander would require before using biological weapons—either tactically or strategically—as anything more than a hopeful addition to conventional weapons, could be obtained without field trials on man or whatever was the chosen target. Such trials would be dangerous, and virtually impossible to conduct in peace time. This objection, to my mind, would make biological agents unattractive except perhaps for purposes of sabotage or as an indiscriminate and uncertain means of producing mass destruction or large scale panic and confusion. The objection applies whether the biological agents were intended to be lethal, and to cause epidemic spread, or whether they were intended to cause transient crippling disease without subsequent dissemination. I speak, of course, as an outsider, but I cannot see how a hard-headed military commander could regard biological agents as potential war-winning weapons. This is not to say that they might not be tried as a gimmick, or as a means of weakening the resistance of the people of an island, such as Britain, to which their effects could be more or less confined. In fact, in a recent television programme on biological weapons, entitled "A Plague on Your Children", an American biological warfare expert, Brigadier General Rothschild, was at pains to point out what an ideal target Britain would present. He did not explain for what purpose, or in what sort of war.

I have taken a long time to reach the question which is the subject of this Symposium because it seems to me that two separate issues are involved. The first concerns whether wars at all are acceptable or inevitable, and the second whether, if wars have to be reckoned with, biological weapons should be used in them.

Much has been said and written about man's peculiar aggressiveness against his own kind, and about the causes of its channelling into war.

So long as nations maintain military machinery as the accepted means of threatening each other wars may not be inevitable, but they are highly probable. The sociological and educational progress required to make war unacceptable to enough people, even in the so-called advanced countries, to reverse this situation is so slow that I have come to think that we cannot reckon on its happening. However, whether one's views about this are optimistic or pessimistic, it is evident that the scale of destruction and misery which result from war depend upon the weapons which are used in fighting. Engineers, chemists and physicists have invented a panoply of fantastic destructiveness, which one might have thought would suffice any military commander; but now the biologists are seriously being called in for the first time, apart from those who devise weapons for psychological warfare. We are told— and doubtless it is true—that other countries are devising biological weapons, and that these may be used against us, so that we should connive at preparations for the defence of this country against them even if we do not go so far as actually to assist. Presumably the biologists in other countries are being told the same. It is emphasized that such preparations provide much information which is useful in peace time, just as part of the justification for the development of new offensive and defensive weapons in other fields is given as their industrial "spin off". It is also admitted that research on methods of defence inevitably requires research on methods of offence, even if there is no present intention of using or developing the latter in this country.

Biologists, just as anyone else, may have opinions about war, but ought they to have opinions about biological weapons as such? Despite the revulsion which many people feel against them, I cannot see that biological weapons pose any greater ethical or moral problem than do other indiscriminate weapons, either to those that make or to those that use them. In fact I doubt whether to someone at the receiving end an attack with such weapons could be more unpleasant than one with napalm or saturation bombing with anti-personnel missiles, which have become everyday events in Vietnam. As I have already implied, I do not think that biological weapons *at their present stage of development* are of great military importance; the problems which they raise are certainly far less urgent than those raised by the nuclear weapons and ballistic missiles which have already been developed. It may well seem illogical to make a fuss about them, unless there are reasons for distinguishing them from other weapons on grounds apart from novelty or sheer beastliness. However, I think that there are such reasons. They apply also to chemical weapons, except that these have not only been tried out successfully but are known to have been developed extensively in the armoury of both the Western and the Eastern Powers.

The first, and perhaps most important, is that people in all countries and politicians in their public pronouncements do make a distinction— even though it may be illogical, and based on an accident of propaganda and of history. The terms of the Geneva Protocol, publicly supported since December 1966 by all the major powers (including the non-signatories Japan and the U.S.A.), forbid the first use of chemical and biological weapons in warfare, even though they do not forbid research on or possession of such weapons. Despite its obscurities, and the tenuousness of any guarantee of observance, the Geneva Protocol provides a specific statement of intention which it has not hitherto been possible to achieve in respect of other weapons.

The second is that investment in biological weapons, though not negligible, is still very small compared with that in conventional and nuclear weapons. The arguments in their favour have been briefly summarized above. One which appears to be finding favour at present— especially in relation to chemical weapons—is that non-lethal forms could provide a humane means of winning wars. Since few persons— at least in peace time—relish the idea of killing people, the claim of humaneness could lead to increased investment in them and could undermine the public antipathy towards them quite rapidly. However, I find it hard to see (and this doubt is confirmed by the example of the use of non-lethal chemical weapons in Vietnam) how such weapons could deter or defeat a determined enemy, except when used as a means of making other weapons more effective. This question requires some hard thinking, and I do not propose to pursue it here.

The third is that much of the research needed to develop biological weapons, or to provide defence against them, is very similar to research which might legitimately be done for peaceful purposes in universities, medical research and public health institutes, and enterprises engaged in the manufacture of vaccines. Examples would be studies of factors controlling the pathogenicity of microbes and their mode of dissemination; of methods for rapid identification and detection; of large scale culture techniques; of preparation of protective vaccines, and so on. Even intensive investigation of exotic highly virulent microbes would be entirely proper in a wholly peaceful world, both on scientific grounds and because of the possibility that sometime, somewhere, they might become disseminated and give rise to serious epidemics such as have ravaged man and his animals in the past. Microbiological research and development become biological weapon research only in so far as techniques are devised for deliberately spreading pathogenic infective agents in war.

The fourth is that because of the enormous potential activity per unit weight of biological weapons quite small factories, or even parts of factories, could suffice to supply the military needs. Apart from the special precautions essential for handling such highly dangerous materials nothing obvious need distinguish such factories from others making antibiotics or microbial vaccines. Consequently inspection to ascertain whether the ingredients for such weapons were being made would present much greater difficulties than in the case of, for example, fissile materials for nuclear weapons.

With these points in mind, I think that it is possible to have an attitude towards biological weapons which could conceivably help towards solving the more important and pressing general problems of disarmament, while allowing us, as biologists, to take a public stand against the diversion of our work to military ends. Admittedly the attitude is largely political, but, as von Clausewitz wrote, "war is nothing more than the continuation of politics by other means". We can help to ensure that the support publicly given to the Geneva Protocol by almost all the national delegations at the General Assembly of the United Nations in December 1966 is strengthened and not eroded. This means that the issues involved must be clearly understood and discussed widely enough to put pressure at home and abroad on the governments of those countries which have not yet ratified the Protocol to do so. Without wishing to minimize the unpleasantness of biological weapons, or the objections to any weapons whose effects are indiscriminate, I think that the most valid reason is that the Geneva Protocol, if not a giant confidence trick, is a real beginning of that limitation of weapons which all countries in the United Nations have declared they wish to seek. Until the difficulties presented by inspection and verification have been got round it will be difficult to extend the Protocol to forbid research on or possession of biological weapons, though states could be encouraged to renounce these for thelselves, as Austria has done. Meanwhile, interpretation of the Geneva Protocol requires clarification at two points. One is whether the prohibition includes crop destroying agents, and the second whether a distinction is to be drawn between lethal and non-lethal agents. To take the second point first, it seems to me that only by making *no* distinction and forbidding all chemical and biological weapons can difficulties of interpretation and the danger of retaliation with weapons of increasing lethability be avoided. For the same reason I think that the use of anti-crop weapons should also be completely prohibited. The argument that tear gas is commonly used for civilian riot control, and that spraying with herbicides is normal agricultural practice, is a red herring. The situations in which they are so used have nothing to do with war, and no one intends to forbid their possession or use in civilian life.

Even if all countries had adhered to the Geneva Protocol allegations of infringement in times of tension or war might still be made, and would require rapid investigation, since the right of retaliation in kind would remain. There should be a recognized organization prepared to do this which would need the willing cooperation of microbiologists. It might be the International Red Cross Organization, or perhaps the World Health Organization because of its accepted expertise in epidemiology and its non-partisan reputation. All this would minimize the danger of the future use of biological weapons, but it would not prevent countries from researching on and preparing such weapons as a precautionary measure to permit retaliation.

The next and more important goal is for all countries to renounce the use of biological weapons altogether. This would imply that no secret research, by government or industry, could be done on potential weapon agents, and that open research on them in scale and content must have a clearly non-military aim. Renunciation of biological weapons could be made soon—and indeed might become much more difficult later—because no country has yet made such a major investment in these weapons as to feel its security threatened by renouncing them as part of a general agreement. It would be furthermore a gesture of mutual confidence, even though a small one, which could lead to other and more important steps towards disarmament in more sensitive areas. However, if the renunciation were made within the next few years, as it should be, it is unlikely that the degree of mutual trust between states would be sufficient to dispense with the need for some means of guaranteeing that the agreement would be observed. Within the Western European Union a working system of inspection covering chemical weapons has been evolved as part of the agreement on ceiling levels for arms production by each member. To extend this from countries which are military allies, but commercial rivals, to all countries would not be easy unless at least a modest degree of mutual confidence between them existed. But unless mutual confidence increases the outlook is bleak indeed; since confidence breeds confidence, and suspicion breeds suspicion, why not make a beginning here where a common interest is involved? The problem of inspection for biological weapons is particularly difficult. A start has been made by the Pugwash movement in conducting voluntary inspections of academic research establishments capable of producing ingredients of such weapons in Sweden, Denmark, Czechoslovakia and Austria. The Stockholm International Peace Research Institute (SIPRI) is currently extending such a voluntary inspection to include commercial firms in various countries. The inspectors who began pessimistic about the possibility were encouraged by the preliminary inspections, and the outlook for this type of control does nor appear entirely hopeless, given sufficient goodwill. A different approach is being undertaken jointly by a Swedish and a Russian microbiologist inder the auspices of SIPRI, which is to investigate the possibility of detecting micro-organisms in minute amounts over areas of permanent snow with a view to testing the feasibility of detecting the liberation of aerosol clouds of microbes hundreds or thousands of miles away, such as would be required for a field test. The feasibility of this depends upon the use of extraordinarily sensitive techniques and on the presence of a negligible background contamination of the air. The project may be hopeless, but at least it will be scientifically valuable and I mention it to illustrate the sorts of approaches which are being made.

I wish to stress that if once all countries had officially abjured biological warfare, with its attendent secrecy, the problems would be much simplified. For example, even statistics of the degree of production or stockpiling of protective clothing and masks, or knowledge of whether military or civilian instruction in their use was being given, could give warning of an impending infringement. Furthermore, a powerful sense of internationalism is growing up among scientists and technologists, who—if secret preparations for biological warfare were begun—would have to be engaged in infringing publicly stated agreements made by their own country. Under such circumstances it is conceivable that open surveillance exercised by scientists themselves— acting, for example, through the International Union for the relevant science—could be important in making infringement much more difficult.

What should be the future of the establishments which have been built up to study and prepare for national defence (and to a greater or lesser degree, offence) in relation to biological warfare? It is important to consider this question, since on the one hand they are likely to have a powerful vested interest in their own continued existence, with the possibility of arguing for this at the top level, and on the other hand they contain skilled teams including chemists, engineers, physicists, pharmacologists, pathologists and microbiologists, etc. possessing very great expertise in the study of microbial pathogens, or aerosol behaviour, of meteorology, and of protective clothing. Much of their work has a direct relation to the problems of civilian life, but it has much less impact on these than it might do if the primary object of the establishments were not to undertake partly classified work for their defence ministries.

I will consider our own establishment, the M.R.E. at Porton Down, and will assume that its own public image of itself is broadly correct. That is, that its function is to study potential offensive agents only in relation to devising means of defence against them; that the great bulk of the original scientific work done there is published; and that most of the scientists take jobs there not only to earn a reasonable salary, but because they are given excellent facilities to study scientifically interesting problems and because they have a genuine belief that their work is important for the military defence of the country. Furthermore, I know that it is willing to help other civilian institutions with advice and the provision of materials and facilities. Nevertheless, in accepting this image I think it necessary to remember that the study of defensive measures may not be so innocent as it might appear if studies of offensive measures and discoveries relating to these are left to our American allies on a reciprocal basis.

I do not, of course, know what classified work goes on at the M.R.E. Let us suppose hypothetically, however, that significant defence advances have been made such as the development of a very effective general purpose gas mask or of a rapid and extremely sensitive method for detecting airborne microbes. Would the revelation of such developments diminish their defensive value? Or might not this actually be increased, by showing that it would be very difficult for one country to steal a march on another in this field?

Assuming that our government is not contemplating becoming engaged in a war within the next few years involving biological weapons—despite the Geneva Protocol—and especially if, as Mr. Fred Mulley's recent proposals to the Disarmament Conference at Geneva suggest, it were meanwhile prepared to make a real effort at the international level to reach agreement to renounce these weapons, I suggest that for a trial period future work carried out at Porton should be declassified. Admittedly work may be done there which could facilitate the devising of more effective biological weapons, and whose development would not be in the interest of this country or of mankind. This may, though less probably, occur also in other research establishments. I can see that there could be a case for not publishing such work unless it was of general theoretical interest, and there would certainly be a case for not pursuing it on anything more than a small experimental scale. The case would not, however, be essentially different at M.R.E. from any other establishment, and the decision would rest with the scientists concerned and the Director (with the concurrence of any advisory council), and would not require the application of the Official Secrets Act. Work on the defence of man and animals against highly virulent and pathogenic organisms could proceed much as at present, and might well be the more effective because collaboration with other workers would be easier and more natural. Of course the results would not be the exclusive property of the Ministry of Defence, but there would be nothing to prevent the armed forces from obtaining advice and making use of them as they wished. Even during the trial period I would like to see at least a part of M.R.E. positively devoted to collaboration with the World Health Organization over problems of mutual interest (of which there are many) or with the Food and Agriculture Organization over such things as the large scale production of micro-organisms as food additives for regions where dietary protein is inadequate. Collaboration of this sort would not only have the advantage of promoting goodwill but could help towards defraying the cost of keeping Porton going.

To make such a gesture would carry some risk, but it would be an act of leadership by this country which could produce quite disproportionate gains by helping to break the deadlock over disarmament. Furthermore, by making the gesture for an initial trial period, without disbanding the teams which have been built up, even the risk would be minimized.

In trying to discuss my subject realistically I hope that I have not set ethics too much to one side. However, to my mind the real test of ethical principles is how they look when applied in practice. If the suggestions which I have made appear half-baked, perhaps members of the Institute of Biology may be able to improve upon them. If more biologists were to give serious thought to the problems of inspection and verification they might find a practical solution. Furthermore, biological weapons cannot be made, or biological warfare conducted, without the help of biologists, and it would be a good thing if the public—which shows signs of growing scepticism about the necessary benefits of scientific advance—were to know that biologists were conscious of their responsibility in this matter.

Discussion

MOORE: Dr. Darling asked for action not just words; I write as one whose job it is to carry out practical conservation measures. He stated that life exists in its own right: I have great sympathy with this concept, but can he advise conservationists on how we should act on this principle in practice? In each case of conflict, whether it is over the protection of a site of scientific value, or concerns restrictions on use of a pesticide, we are always up against the fact that man *is* the ecological dominant. Should man always have priority? How should Dr. Darling's concept affect our activities?

FRASER DARLING: It would be fatuous, as well as futile, to expect man to allow his species to be decimated by diseases caused by insect or helminthic vectors in deference to a concept of reverence for life of all kinds. But even acts of self preservation demand a sense of responsibility in policies which may lay man open to such diseases. Few can be so ingenuous as to imagine that an irrigation scheme in Africa is designed to cure starvation, but such a scheme will certainly spread the snail which is intermediate host to the schistosome. Man is constantly putting himself into situations in which his backlash against other forms of life will be more severe. In such situations man's discipline in forethought should be more severe. In the matter of the sanctity of a site of scientific or aesthetic value I think the issue is clearer: we have no right to act expediently or to deprive our own posterity.

BUSVINE: I must take issue with Dr. Fraser Darling on his examples of alleged harm done by controlling arthropod pests. Malaria control has succeeded in actually *eradicating* the disease from countries where 1,000 million people were formerly at risk, merely by insecticidal control of the anopheline vector. In no case has this resulted in the appearance of a new anopheline vector, though, of course, such campaigns naturally focus attention on the small numbers of refractory anophelines, such as those which breed in epiphytes (to which, I suppose he refers).

As regards the red mite in orchards, this case is nearer the mark. It is not a new pest, but an old one favoured by insecticides used (successfully) against other orchard pests, but which happen to kill off predators and parasites of the red mites. The relevance of the tse-tse is not clear; we are very far from doing serious harm to this scourge of tropical Africa.

133

FRASER DARLING: I was thinking of Colin Pittendrigh's work in South America in the 1940's. If I remember aright, control of one anopheline allowed another breeding at a different elevation to bring about diurnal infection. Shade control was also concerned. My allusion to red mite pointed to a non-ecological method of control which was both ineffective and possibly unethical. Our right to self preservation by control measures is not in opposition to a respect for life of other creatures, but I think we could say that ecological forethought and ecological methods in control measures could prevent a lot of needless killing and of upsets in natural communities. The distribution of tse-tse can be linked quite often with human mismanagement of land, for example, bush encroachment following an inept fire regime; and removal of tse-tse may lead to serious soil erosion and habitat deterioration if grazing of domesticated animals is thereafter not very carefully controlled. Here again, neglect of ecological forethought can well be unethical when the knowledge is available.

HEDEN: First I would like to compliment Dr. Humphrey on going over this extremely difficult ground so carefully and at the same time providing so many constructive proposals. One of the major difficulties is embodied in Leo Szilard's version of Einstein's comment when the latter was asked about his opinion of the League of Nation's disarmament conference in 1926. "What would you think", Einstein asked, "about a meeting of a town council which is convened because an increasing number of people are knifed to death each night in drunken brawls, and which proceeds to discuss just how long and how sharp shall be the knife that the inhabitants of the city may be per-permitted to carry?"

I share most of Dr. Humphrey's views, except that I would perhaps be slightly more guarded in passing the judgement that biological weapons have a low military importance at their present stage of development. I would have felt that this required a distinction between strategic and tactical use, and particularly between overt and covert use. I tend to agree with Dr. Humphrey when it comes to overt strategic use. In this system weapons of a reliability and versatility required by the military men may perhaps not yet be available. As I see it, it is consequently in this area where efforts towards disarmament on an inter-governmental level may pay off. It is the tactical and covert use which worries me, because the weapons exist and adequate controls, with inspection procedures which would be a part of inter-governmental agreements, seem impossible. Even field trials, which Dr. Humphrey regards as virtually impossible to carry out in peace time, would be extremely hard to detect if carried out on foreign soil. How could we then limit the hazards of covert use in the type of guerilla-counter insurgency situations which seem to be disturbingly common? I will not complicate the issue by discussing the moral value of different reactions to opressive rule, but I would like to ask Dr. Humphrey if he thinks that there is any better alternative—if we want to see a limitation of biological weapons—than the establishment of an international code of ethics, an equivalent to the Hippocratic oath.

HUMPHREY: The drawback to establishing an international code of ethics is that it would be very difficult to enforce. The strength of professional codes of conduct, such as that of the medical profession (which is derived from the Hippocratic oath even if this is not sworn) or of the legal profession is that they are enforced by chartered bodies which can deprive of their professional status those who infringe the codes. The codes have quite as firm an economic as an ethical basis, and are required to protect potentially powerful groups from the suspicion with which their power would otherwise be regarded by the rest of society. Scientists, *qua* scientists, do indeed form a powerful sector of society, but they are very heterogeneous, and in the main, employees of other bodies. They have not for long enough enjoyed as a group the self-employed and largely independent status of the two professions which I mentioned. Nevertheless, the establishment of a code of conduct would indeed provide one possible approach, and should be pursued. It might be enforceable by the learned societies, given sufficient lead perhaps by the International Council of Scientific Unions, to which many of them are indirectly affiliated. But ICSU and the societies themselves would have to change their spots before this happened.

WOODRUFF: If I might be the devil's advocate, I should like to put to Dr. Humphrey a defence of biological weapons which is often made, namely, that they are cheap and hence available to smaller or weaker nations.

HUMPHREY: I agree that biological weapons are potentially cheap, though this does not—to my mind—negate the military disadvantages which I mentioned. Furthermore, except possibly at the level of sabotage I doubt whether their employment would give a small or a poor country the edge over a larger and richer one because defence against them would be expensive, and there would be a high probability of escalation in reprisals. In fact I suspect that the interest of the U.S.A. in biological and, especially, chemical weapons derives partly from the idea that these could be used in limited counter-insurgency operations against a hidden and scattered enemy.

LE GROS CLARK: Biologists must have their own ethics. Those who are microbiologists know when work is for offensive purposes and they should decide not to participate in such work.

HUMPHREY: If Professor Le Gros Clarke's definition of offensive is something like that which I gave, that microbiological research and development become biological warfare research only insofar as techniques are devised for deliberately spreading pathogenic infective agents in war, I agree with him that it should be obvious to microbiologists what they are up to, and they should not do it. However, the argument which was put across intensively in the U.S.A. in the "Operation Blue Skies" propaganda campaign, namely that biological weapons could provide a "humane" way of winning wars, seems to have convinced at least some of those involved in producing these weapons in the U.S.A., and it needs examining carefully. If it is wrong it needs refuting. My own view is that the presumption that "humane" weapons (used humanely) could win a war is based on the conviction of the users that their aims are wholly just and that if their opponents could be stopped in their tracks long enough to reflect, they would realize how mistaken they are. This is not how the opposing aims are viewed once a war has begun.

EBLING: I agree most strongly with Professor Le Gros Clark. The scientist has a responsibility in direct proportion to his knowledge and understanding and it cannot be passed to others. Francis Bacon, at the very birth of the modern scientific age, understood that science was too dangerous to be pursued merely for itself without reference to its purpose "which is the benefit and relief of the state and society of man; for otherwise all manner of knowledge becometh malign".

WYATT: It may be necessary to grow large quantities of pathogenic organisms for peaceful uses. Jonas Salk chose the Mahoney Type I strain of polio virus for his vaccine, knowing that it was one of the most pathogenic isolated. It may therefore be extremely difficult to distinguish legitimate research from covert work on biological weapons.

MASON: My dominant impression gathered from the symposium is that almost all the things discussed hinge on the fact that the world has grown very small and very full of people. As a modern poet has put it: "What we do best is breed". But whereas, previously, we were breeding with a low survival rate now we are breeding with a high survival rate without stopping to consider world implications of what we do. We must begin to think globally (as people as well as scientists), and try to hammer out new, commonsense ethics to fit new situations in a shrinking environment.

Two practical possibilities of limiting population that biologists might discuss are firstly, fiscal methods, such as removing spinster and bachelor taxes, diminishing and phasing our family allowances, revising our status attitudes to homosexuals and other non-breeding groups. (Existing children would not of course be penalized). Secondly, techniques of sex control as soon as we have them should be tried out in pilot schemes with consenting couples and if, as I would guess, the trend of choice is toward boy babies, at least at the beginning, the techniques could be widely used to reduce the number of potential future mothers.

BLACKHAM: I should like to add to the Symposium a note on the theoretical perspective. Eighteenth century philosophers looked forward confidently to a science of "human nature". Moral philosophers before this generation assumed that psychology was a main ingredient in ethics; but a professor of psychology said to me recently that for his students Freud was as remote as Aristotle—and remember Freud was a neurologist looking for a "scientific" theory of human behaviour. Old style intuitive theories about human behaviour and human nature, on which academic discussion of ethics used to depend until lately, have disappeared. A "science of human nature" seems to be out of the question today and the "concept of human nature" is a philosophical ghost. Only theologians still travel along traditional paths. Does this matter? Is any other conceptual control or result needed or will linguistic analysis and specific research programmes take care of all that matters?

TOWERS: But surely we must have confidence in our ability to arrive at valid conclusions, as the result and purpose of the analysis that is now proceeding everywhere? It seems to me that mankind today is engaged on a kind of "collective psychoanalysis"—but without an analyst standing by to help with support and interpretation when things get difficult. We must find the answers for ourselves by free exchange of experiences and ideas. It is surely right to hope and trust that valid conclusions will emerge in due course, if we only think and work hard enough in a co-operative spirit.

O'DONOGHUE: During the Symposium we have had a succession of intelligent and lucid papers but, alas, I at least am still not sure what ethics are. I do know some things they are *not*. A previous contributor suggested that ethics are things used by the elderly for bamboozling the young; her remarks caused a certain uneasiness but little else. This lack of reaction is a pity for her point was a valuable one—we prostitute the term ethics by applying it to cover our own uncertainty, inadequacy and fear, using it in any situation where we could do with a little spurious authority. Whatever ethics actually are, it is a marked disservice to them when we claim the support of God, tradition, Parliament and so forth, for our whims, prejudices and selfish desires.

As far as professional codes of ethics (architectural, legal, medical, etc.) are concerned, it is my view that when you strip away the trade union regulations that masquerade there you are left with nothing but special applications of general ethical principles. I very much doubt whether regulations applied to certain trades should be dignified as ethical codes, any more than that we should claim ethical foundations for unconvincing arguments with the young.

In discussing man's responsibility for the environment, Dr. Fraser Darling writes of a "reverence for life". I am most impressed, indeed moved, by his approach, and I agree with virtually everything that he writes. However, my mind is too limited to accept his basic reasoning. He rejected the petty, practical reasons for conservation but such small, graspable points are the stuff of conservation (and, indeed, of all ethical matters) for me, even if the point is merely that we cannot know the full consequences of our actions and had therefore best go carefully.

I suspect that ethics are really a series of entirely practical checks and rules which help to ensure our stability and survival as a communal species. The fact that we often do not fully understand the significance or the survival value of these rules encourages a religious, mystical aura, but they are nevertheless essentially of vital, practical importance. Individually it is often profitable to flout them, but only for a while, only while most other individuals observe them; avoidance of ethical behaviour is a short-term view, adoption a long-term one. It follows that ethics are to serve, not to stultify, society, the right to make decisions being limited by uncertainty as to what will constitute the best service, and by the consequent realization that no ethical decision can be sacrosanct and irrevocable. There are, of course, dangers inherent in this view, but similar penalties are incurred when the practical basis and ends are forgotten, or allowed to founder in a welter of ethereal discussion. To me, then, ethics are a biological and social matter common to our species: local and other special applications abound but there is really only one ethical code. Although biologists should be deeply concerned with ethical problems, we waste time and dangerously confuse issues if we seek to set up a unique code for our or any other professional group.

Subject Index